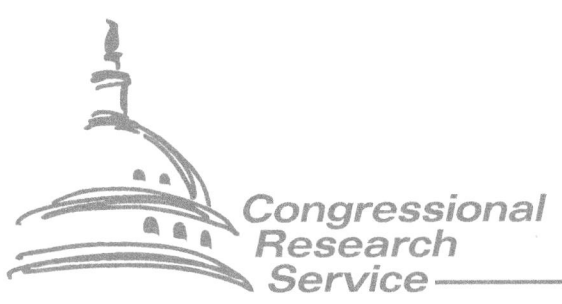

Congressional
Research
Service

Medicaid Disproportionate Share Hospital Payments

Alison Mitchell
Analyst in Health Care Financing

December 18, 2012

Congressional Research Service

7-5700

www.crs.gov

R42865

Summary

The Medicaid statute requires states to make disproportionate share hospital (DSH) payments to hospitals treating large numbers of low-income patients. This provision is intended to recognize the disadvantaged financial situation of those hospitals because low-income patients are more likely to be uninsured or Medicaid enrollees. Hospitals often do not receive payment for services rendered to uninsured patients, and Medicaid provider payment rates are generally lower than the rates paid by Medicare and private insurance.

As with most Medicaid expenditures, the federal government reimburses states for a portion of their Medicaid DSH expenditures based on each state's federal medical assistance percentage (FMAP). While most federal Medicaid funding is provided on an open-ended basis, federal Medicaid DSH funding is capped. Each state receives an annual DSH allotment, which is the maximum amount of federal matching funds that each state is permitted to claim for Medicaid DSH payments. In FY2012, federal DSH allotments totaled $11.3 billion.

The health insurance coverage provisions of the Patient Protection and Affordable Care Act (ACA, P.L. 111-148 as amended) are expected to reduce the number of uninsured individuals in the United States, which means there should be less need for Medicaid DSH payments. As a result, the ACA included a provision directing the Secretary of the Department of Health and Human Services to make aggregate reductions in federal Medicaid DSH allotments for each year from FY2014 to FY2020. The Middle Class Tax Relief and Job Creation Act of 2012 (P.L. 112-96) extended the DSH reductions to FY2021. The Supreme Court's decision regarding the ACA Medicaid expansion does not impact these DSH reduction amounts, but states' decisions about implementing the ACA Medicaid expansion could impact the allocation of the DSH reductions across states.

While there are some federal requirements that states must follow in defining DSH hospitals and calculating DSH payments, for the most part, states are provided significant flexibility. One way the federal government restricts states' Medicaid DSH payments is that the federal statute limits the amount of DSH payments for Institutions for Mental Disease and other mental health facilities.

Since Medicaid DSH allotments were implemented in FY1993, total Medicaid DSH expenditures (i.e., including federal and state expenditures) have remained relatively stable. Over this same period of time, total Medicaid DSH expenditures as a percentage of total Medicaid medical assistance expenditures (i.e., including both federal and state expenditures but excluding expenditures for administrative activities) dropped from 13% to 4%.

This report provides an overview of Medicaid DSH. It includes a description of the rules delineating how state DSH allotments are calculated and the exceptions to the rules, how DSH hospitals are defined, and how DSH payments are calculated. The DSH allotment section includes information about how the ACA DSH reductions may be allocated among the states, and the possible implications of the Supreme Court's decision regarding the ACA Medicaid expansion. The DSH expenditures section shows the trends in DSH spending and explains variation in states' DSH expenditures. Finally, the basic requirements for state DSH reports and independently certified audits are also outlined.

Contents

Figures

Tables

Appendixes

Contacts

Introduction

Medicaid is a federal-state program providing medical assistance for low-income individuals.[1] Historically, Medicaid eligibility has generally been limited to low-income children, pregnant women, parents of dependent children, the elderly, and individuals with disabilities; however, recent changes will soon add coverage for individuals under the age of 65 with income up to 133% of the federal poverty level.[2]

Participation in Medicaid is voluntary for states, though all states, the District of Columbia, and territories[3] choose to participate. In order to participate in Medicaid, the federal government requires states to cover certain mandatory populations and benefits, but the federal government also allows states to cover optional populations and services.[4] Due to this flexibility, there is substantial variation among the states in terms of factors such as Medicaid eligibility, covered benefits, and provider payment rates.

Medicaid is jointly financed by the federal government and the states. States incur Medicaid costs by making payments to service providers (e.g., for doctor visits) and performing administrative activities (e.g., making eligibility determinations), and the federal government reimburses states for a share of these costs.[5] The federal government's share of a state's expenditures for most Medicaid services is called the federal medical assistance percentage (FMAP).[6] The FMAP varies by state and is inversely related to each state's per capita income. For FY2013, FMAP rates range from 50% (14 states) to 73% (Mississippi), and, on average, the federal contribution covers about 57% of the total cost of Medicaid in a typical year.

The Medicaid statute requires that states make disproportionate share hospital (DSH) payments to hospitals treating large numbers of low-income patients.[7] This provision is intended to recognize

---

[1] For more information about the Medicaid program, see CRS Report RL33202, *Medicaid: A Primer*, by Elicia J. Herz.

[2] The Patient Protection and Affordable Care Act (ACA, P.L. 111-148 as amended) establishes 133% of federal poverty level (FPL) based on modified adjusted gross income (MAGI) as the new mandatory minimum Medicaid income eligibility level. The law also specifies that an income disregard in the amount of 5% FPL will be deducted from an individual's income when determining Medicaid eligibility based on MAGI. Thus, the effective upper income eligibility threshold for individuals in this new eligibility group will be 138% FPL. On November 21, 2011, President Obama signed into law P.L. 112-56, which changes the definition of income to include non-taxable Social Security in the definition of MAGI.

[3] The territories are American Samoa, Guam, the Commonwealth of the Northern Mariana Islands, Puerto Rico, and the Virgin Islands.

[4] On June 28, 2012, the United States Supreme Court issued its decision in *National Federation of Independent Business v. Sebelius*, finding that the federal government cannot terminate current Medicaid program federal matching funds if a state refuses to implement the Medicaid expansion required by ACA. If a state accepts the new ACA Medicaid expansion funds, it must abide by the new expansion coverage rules, but, based on the Court's opinion, it appears that a state can refuse to participate in the expansion without losing any of its current federal Medicaid matching funds.

[5] For an overview of Medicaid financing issues, see CRS Report R42640, *Medicaid Financing and Expenditures*, by Alison Mitchell.

[6] For more information about the FMAP rate, see CRS Report RL32950, *Medicaid: The Federal Medical Assistance Percentage (FMAP)*, by Alison Mitchell and Evelyne P. Baumrucker.

[7] The Medicare program also makes DSH payments. Medicaid and Medicare DSH hospital payments are similar in that the major basis for designating hospitals to receive payments is the proportion of services provided to low-income patients. However, Medicaid and Medicare have different criteria for identifying DSH hospitals, and the programs have different calculations for determining DSH payment amounts. For FY2012, Medicare DSH payments are estimated to (continued...)

---

the disadvantaged financial situation of such hospitals because low-income patients are more likely to be uninsured or Medicaid enrollees. Hospitals often do not receive payment for services rendered to uninsured patients, and Medicaid provider payment rates are generally lower than the rates paid by Medicare and private insurance.

While most federal Medicaid funding is provided on an open-ended basis, federal Medicaid DSH funding is capped. Each state receives an annual federal DSH allotment, which is the maximum amount of federal matching funds that each state can claim for Medicaid DSH payments. In FY2012, the federal DSH allotments to states totaled $11.3 billion.

This report provides an overview of Medicaid DSH, including how state DSH allotments are calculated and the exceptions to the DSH allotments calculation; how DSH hospitals are defined and how DSH payments to hospitals are calculated; trends in DSH spending; variation in states' DSH expenditures; and requirements outlining the basics requirements for state DSH reports and independently certified audits. The DSH allotment section includes information about how the ACA DSH reductions will be allocated among the states, and the potential implications of the Supreme Court's decision in *National Federation of Independent Business v. Sebelius*.

Background: Medicaid DSH

Medicaid DSH payments were established in the Omnibus Budget Reconciliation Act of 1981 (OBRA 1981, P.L. 97-35) when the methodology for Medicaid payment rates to hospitals was amended.[8] Prior to OBRA 1981, state Medicaid programs were required to reimburse hospitals on a reasonable cost basis (as defined under Medicare) unless the state had approval to use an alternate payment method.[9] This law deleted the reasonable cost methodology and transferred the responsibility for determining Medicaid payment rates to the states.

A new provision required Medicaid hospital payment rates to take into account the situation of hospitals that serve a disproportionate number of "low income patients with special needs."[10] This requirement established the Medicaid DSH payments.

The inclusion of this Medicaid DSH provision in OBRA 1981 recognized that hospitals serving a disproportionate share of low income patients are particularly dependent on Medicaid payments because low income patients are mostly Medicaid enrollees and uninsured individuals.[11] Hospitals often do not receive payment for services rendered to uninsured patients, and Medicaid provider payment rates are generally lower than the rates paid by Medicare and private insurance.

(...continued)

be $10.8 billion. (Congressional Budget Office, *Medicare – March 2012 Baseline*, March 13, 2012.)

[8] The DSH provision was included in a package of provisions referred to as the "Boren amendment" after its sponsor, Senator David Boren from Oklahoma.

[9] The Secretary of Health and Human Services could approve an alternate system only if the Secretary determined that (1) a reasonable cost was paid (though the state could develop its own methods and standards for determining what was reasonable) and (2) the reasonable cost did not exceed the amount which would be determined reasonable under Medicare.

[10] Section 1902(a)(13)(A)(iv) of the Social Security Act.

[11] Conf. Rept. 97-208.

States Slow to Implement DSH Programs

While the requirement to make DSH payments was originally established in 1981, many states did not make DSH payments throughout the 1980s. As a result, other federal laws were enacted with provisions aimed at getting states to make DSH payments. For instance, a provision in the Omnibus Budget Reconciliation Act of 1986 (P.L. 99-509) was aimed at supporting state flexibility to make DSH payments. Also, the Omnibus Budget Reconciliation Act of 1987 (P.L. 100-203) required states to submit a Medicaid state plan amendment[12] describing their DSH policies and establishing certain minimum qualifying standards and payments.

Sharp Increase in DSH Expenditures

DSH payments quickly became a significant portion of Medicaid spending in the early 1990s. DSH expenditures (including federal and state expenditures) grew from $1.0 billion in FY1990 to $17.4 billion in FY1992. As a percent of total Medicaid medical assistance expenditures (i.e., including federal and state spending and excluding expenditures for administrative activities), DSH expenditures grew from 1.3% of total Medicaid medical assistance expenditures in FY1990 to 15.0% in FY1992 (see **Table 1**).

Table 1. Total DSH Expenditures and Total DSH Expenditures as a Percentage of Total Medicaid Medical Assistance Expenditures

FY1990 to FY1992

	DSH Expenditures (in billions)	Percent Increase	DSH Expenditures as a % of Medical Assistance Expenditures
FY1990	$1.0	NA	1.3%
FY1991	$4.7	370.0%	5.2%
FY1992	$17.4	270.2%	15.0%

Source: Payments estimated by the Urban Institute.

Notes: Total DSH expenditures include both federal and state spending on DSH payments. Total Medicaid medical assistance expenditures include federal and state spending and exclude Medicaid spending on administrative activities.

DSH = Disproportionate Share Hospital.

The significant increase in DSH expenditures was not attributed to the laws enacted by Congress. Instead, the growth in Medicaid expenditures coincided with states' increased use of provider taxes and donations to help finance the state share of Medicaid expenditures.[13] DSH payments

---

[12] A Medicaid State Plan is a contract between a state and the federal government describing how that state administers its Medicaid program, and a state is required to submit a state plan amendment when the state intends to change its Medicaid program.

[13] In the mid-1980s, states began using provider taxes along with provider donations to help finance Medicaid. Essentially, Medicaid providers would donate funds or agree to be taxed, and the revenue from these taxes and donations would be used to finance a portion of the state's share of Medicaid expenditures. Some states were borrowing funds from Medicaid providers in order to draw down federal funds and increase Medicaid payment rates to the same providers that had paid taxes or donated funds. The providers were often fully reimbursed for the cost of their (continued...)

were a popular mechanism for returning provider taxes or donations to hospitals. Medicaid payments for regular inpatient rates were subject to federal upper payment limits, but DSH payments were uncapped and did not need to be tied to specific Medicaid enrollees or services. As a result, states could increase DSH payments by any amount, tax away the state share of the increased DSH payments through provider taxes, and thus draw down unlimited federal funds.

Limits on DSH Payments

This dramatic growth in DSH expenditures again prompted congressional action. The Medicaid Voluntary Contribution and Provider-Specific Tax Amendments of 1991 (P.L. 102-234) established ceilings on federal Medicaid DSH funding for each state.[14] Since FY1993, each state has had its own DSH limit, which is referred to as a "DSH allotment."

DSH Allotments

While most federal Medicaid funding is provided on an open-ended basis, certain types of federal Medicaid funding, such as federal DSH funding, are capped. Each state[15] receives an annual DSH allotment, which is the maximum amount of federal matching funds a state is permitted to claim for Medicaid DSH payments.[16]

The original state DSH allotments provided in FY1993 were based on each state's FY1992 DSH payments. In FY1992, some states provided relatively more DSH payments to hospitals, and, as a result, these states locked in relatively higher Medicaid DSH allotments. Other states made relatively fewer DSH payments, and these states locked in relatively lower DSH allotments.

This disparity still remains to some extent in current DSH allotments because DSH allotments are not distributed according to a formula based on the number of DSH hospitals in a state or the amount of hospital services these hospitals provide to low-income patients. However, over time, the disparity in DSH allotments was reduced by providing larger annual increases to DSH allotments for states that initially made fewer DSH payments and limiting the growth of DSH allotments for states that initially provided relatively more DSH payments.

The methodology for calculating states' annual DSH allotments has changed a number of times over the years. A history of the DSH allotment calculations is provided in **Appendix A**.

(...continued)

tax payment or donation. For more information about Medicaid provider taxes and donations, see CRS Report RS22843, *Medicaid Provider Taxes*, by Alison Mitchell.

[14] Also, the Medicaid Voluntary Contribution and Provider-Specific Tax Amendments (P.L. 102-234) restricted the use of provider donations in financing Medicaid to extremely limited situations and limited states' ability to draw down federal Medicaid matching funds with provider tax revenue.

[15] State is defined as the 50 states and the District of Columbia. DSH allotments are not provided for the five territories (i.e., America Samoa, Commonwealth of the Northern Mariana Islands, Guam, Puerto Rico, and the Virgin Islands). (Section 1923(f)(9) of the Social Security Act).

[16] Each state's regular FMAP rate is used to determine the federal share of DSH payments.

Currently, states' Medicaid DSH allotments are based on each state's prior year DSH allotment. Specifically, a state's DSH allotment is the higher of (1) a state's FY2004 DSH allotment[17] or (2) the prior year's DSH allotment increased by the percentage change in the consumer price index for all urban consumers (CPI-U) for the prior fiscal year. In FY2012, Louisiana was the only state that continued to receive its FY2004 DSH allotment.

In addition, each state's allotment can be no more than the greater of the prior year's allotment or 12% of its total Medicaid medical assistance expenditures (i.e., including federal and state spending and excluding expenditures for administrative activities) during the fiscal year.[18] This rule is referred to as the "12% limit".[19] This means the federal share of DSH expenditures cannot be more than 12% of each state's total Medicaid medical assistance expenditures. In addition, federal regulations specify that aggregate DSH payments, including federal and state expenditures, should not be more than 12% of the total amount of Medicaid medical assistance expenditures for all 50 states and the District of Columbia.[20] This national limit is not an absolute cap but a target.[21] The national DSH payment limit is different from the 12% limit on state DSH allotments because the 12% national payment limit restricts both federal and state spending while the 12% limit for allotments caps only federal spending.

Due to the "12% limit" for state DSH allotments, the Centers for Medicare & Medicaid Services (CMS) must publish preliminary DSH allotments before the start of the fiscal year based on estimated Medicaid expenditures. Then, after the fiscal year has ended, CMS uses actual expenditure data to calculate final DSH allotments.

CMS calculates annual allotments and publishes them in the *Federal Register*. The most recent *Federal Register* notice[22] included final DSH allotments for FY2010 and FY2011 and preliminary DSH allotments for FY2012. The federal DSH allotments for these years are shown in **Table 2**.

---

[17] The Medicare Prescription Drug, Improvement, and Modernization Act of 2003 (MMA, P.L. 108-173) addressed the drop in DSH allotments for many states from FY2002 to FY2003 by providing a 16% increase in DSH allotments for states in FY2004. If a state's FY2004 DSH allotment is higher than the DSH allotment calculated under the pre-MMA calculation, then the state has received that higher DSH allotment amount since FY2004.

[18] Section 1923(f)(3)(B) of the Social Security Act.

[19] When DSH allotments were first implemented, a state with DSH expenditures greater than 12% of its total Medicaid medical assistance expenditures were classified as "high-DSH" states, and "high-DSH" states did not receive annual increases to their DSH allotment.

[20] 42 C.F.R. § 447.297.

[21] This means if a state receives a federal DSH allotment equal to 12% of its total Medicaid medical assistance expenditures and the state uses all of its federal DSH allotment, then with the state matching funds, the state would provide DSH payments in excess of 12% of its total Medicaid medical assistance expenditures. As a result, the national DSH target could be surpassed. However, in FY2011, DSH payments were well below the national DSH target with total DSH payments (i.e., including federal and state expenditures) amounting to 4.2% of total Medicaid medical assistance expenditures (i.e., including federal and state expenditures but excluding administrative services).

[22] Department of Health and Human Services' Centers for Medicare & Medicaid Services, "Medicaid Program: Disproportionate Share Hospital Allotments and Institutions for Mental Diseases Disproportionate Share Hospital Limits for FYs 2010, 2011, and Preliminary FY 2012 Disproportionate Share Hospital Allotments and Limits ," 77 *Federal Register* 43301, July 24, 2012.

Table 2. DSH Allotments for FY2010, FY2011, and FY2012

($ in millions)

State	FY2010[a]			FY2011	FY2012
	Regular DSH Allotment	ARRA Temporary DSH Increase	Final DSH Allotment	Final DSH Allotment	Preliminary DSH Allotment
Alabama	$302.4	$15.3	$317.7	$307.5	$314.9
Alaska[b]	20.0	1.0	21.0	20.4	20.9
Arizona	99.6	5.0	104.6	101.3	103.7
Arkansas[b]	42.4	2.1	44.6	43.1	44.2
California	1,078.0	54.6	1,132.6	1,096.3	1,122.7
Colorado	91.0	4.6	95.6	92.5	94.7
Connecticut	196.7	10.0	206.6	200.0	204.8
Delaware[b]	8.9	0.5	9.4	9.1	9.3
District of Columbia	60.2	3.0	63.3	61.3	62.7
Florida	196.7	10.0	206.6	200.0	204.8
Georgia	264.3	13.4	277.7	268.8	275.2
Hawaii[c]	10.0	0.0	10.0	10.0	10.0
Idaho[b]	16.2	0.8	17.0	16.4	16.8
Illinois	211.4	10.7	222.1	215.0	220.2
Indiana	210.2	10.6	220.8	213.8	218.9
Iowa[b]	38.7	2.0	40.7	39.4	40.3
Kansas	40.6	2.1	42.6	41.3	42.2
Kentucky	142.6	7.2	149.8	145.0	148.5
Louisiana	732.0	37.1	769.0	732.0	732.0
Maine	103.3	5.2	108.5	105.0	107.5
Maryland	75.0	3.8	78.8	76.3	78.1
Massachusetts	299.9	15.2	315.1	305.0	312.3
Michigan	260.6	13.2	273.8	265.0	271.4
Minnesota[b]	73.4	3.7	77.2	74.7	76.5
Mississippi	150.0	7.6	157.6	152.5	156.2
Missouri	465.9	23.6	489.5	473.8	485.2
Montana[b]	11.2	0.6	11.7	11.4	11.6
Nebraska[b]	27.8	1.4	29.2	28.3	29.0
Nevada	45.5	2.3	47.8	46.3	47.4
New Hampshire	157.4	8.0	165.4	160.1	164.0
New Jersey	633.0	32.0	665.1	643.8	659.3
New Mexico[b]	20.0	1.0	21.0	20.4	20.9

State	FY2010[a]			FY2011	FY2012
	Regular DSH Allotment	ARRA Temporary DSH Increase	Final DSH Allotment	Final DSH Allotment	Preliminary DSH Allotment
New York	1,579.5	80.0	1,659.5	1,606.4	1,644.9
North Carolina	290.1	14.7	304.8	295.0	302.1
North Dakota[b]	9.4	0.5	9.9	9.6	9.8
Ohio	399.5	20.2	419.7	406.3	416.0
Oklahoma[b]	35.6	1.8	37.4	36.2	37.1
Oregon	44.5	2.3	46.8	45.3	46.4
Pennsylvania	551.9	27.9	579.9	561.3	574.8
Rhode Island	63.9	3.2	67.2	65.0	66.6
South Carolina	322.1	16.3	338.4	327.5	335.4
South Dakota[b]	10.9	0.5	11.4	11.0	11.3
Tennessee[c]	305.5	0.0	305.5	305.5	123.6
Texas	940.3	47.6	987.9	956.3	979.3
Utah[b]	19.3	1.0	20.3	19.6	20.1
Vermont	22.1	1.1	23.2	22.5	23.0
Virginia	86.2	4.4	90.5	87.6	89.7
Washington	181.9	9.2	191.1	185.0	189.5
West Virginia	66.4	3.4	69.7	67.5	69.1
Wisconsin[b]	93.0	4.7	97.7	94.5	96.8
Wyoming[b]	0.2	0.0	0.2	0.2	0.2
Total	**$11,107.0**	**$546.3**	**11,653.3**	**$11,278.0**	**$11,341.6**

Source: Department of Health and Human Services, "Medicaid Program: Disproportionate Share Hospital Allotments and Institutions for Mental Diseases Disproportionate Share Hospital Limits for FYs 2010, 2011, and Preliminary FY 2012 Disproportionate Share Hospital Allotments and Limits ," 77 *Federal Register* 43301, July 24, 2012.

Notes: DSH allotments are different from DSH payments. Allotments reflect the maximum amount of federal DSH funding available to states, and DSH payments are the amounts paid to hospitals.

FY2010 was the last year the ARRA temporary DSH increase was available to states.

ARRA = American Recovery and Reinvestment Act.

a. States' "Final DSH Allotment" for FY2010 is the combination of the "Regular DSH Allotment" column and the "ARRA Temporary DSH Increase" column.

b. These states are low DSH states. In the past, low DSH states received higher annual percentage increases to their DSH allotments than the non-low DSH states. Currently, low DSH and other states receive the same annual percentage increases to their DSH allotments.

c. Hawaii and Tennessee have special statutory arrangements that specify the DSH allotments for each state.

Exceptions for Certain States

While most states' DSH allotments are determined as described above, the DSH allotments for some states is determined by an alternative method. In the past, low DSH states received higher annual percentage increases to their DSH allotments, but currently low DSH states receive the same annual percentage increases to DSH allotments as other states. Also, Hawaii and Tennessee have special statutory arrangements for the determination of their respective DSH allotments.

Low DSH States

Special rules for low DSH states were initially established by the Medicare, Medicaid, and SCHIP Benefits Improvement and Protection Act of 2000 (BIPA, incorporated into the Consolidated Appropriations Act of 2001, P.L. 106-554).[23] Subsequently, the Medicare Prescription Drug, Improvement, and Modernization Act of 2003 (MMA, P.L. 108-173) amended the definition of low DSH state, and this definition continues to apply today.

States designated as low DSH states were provided greater annual increases to their DSH allotments in order to remove some of the inequities from the initial FY1993 state DSH allotments, which were based on states' DSH expenditures in FY1992. However, increasing DSH allotments does not necessarily mean states will increase their DSH payments. The increased DSH allotments provide states with access to additional federal DSH funding if the states choose to use it.

Under the MMA definition, a low DSH state is defined as a state with FY2000 DSH expenditures greater than 0% but less that 3% of its total Medicaid medical assistance expenditures (i.e., including federal and state expenditures and excluding expenditures for administrative activities) for FY2000. States determined to be low DSH states in FY2004 continue to be low DSH states regardless of their DSH expenditures in years after FY2000.

Sixteen states qualified as low DSH states under the MMA definition, and they continue to be defined as low DSH states. These states are Alaska, Arkansas, Delaware, Idaho, Iowa, Minnesota, Montana, Nebraska, New Mexico, North Dakota, Oklahoma, Oregon, South Dakota, Utah, Wisconsin, and Wyoming.

Each year, from FY2004 through FY2008, low DSH states received a 16% increase to their DSH allotments to increase their DSH allotments relative to other states.[24] For FY2009 and subsequent years, low DSH states receive DSH allotments equal to the prior year's allotment increased by the percent change in CPI-U for the previous fiscal year, which is the same adjustment that non-low DSH states receive.

---

[23] BIPA defined extremely low DSH states as those for which FY1999 total DSH payments (federal and state shares) were greater than zero but less than 1% of the state's total Medicaid medical assistance expenditures (i.e., the federal and state share of Medicaid expenditures excluding administrative expenditures). (Section 1923(f)(5)(A) of the Social Security Act.)

[24] Section 1923(f)(5)(B) of the Social Security Act.

Hawaii and Tennessee

Tennessee and Hawaii operate their state Medicaid programs under Section 1115 research and demonstration waivers,[25] which allow the Secretary of Health and Human Services (HHS) to waive various provisions of Medicaid law. Both states received waivers from making Medicaid DSH payments (among other things), and these states did not receive DSH allotments from FY1998 to FY2006. However, since FY2007, these two states received DSH allotments by special statutory authority provided through multiple laws.[26] **Table 3** shows the federal DSH funding available to Hawaii and Tennessee from FY2007 to FY2014.

Hawaii

Hawaii's DSH allotment was set at $10 million for each of FY2007 through FY2011. Under the Patient Protection and Affordable Care Act (ACA, P.L. 111-148 as amended), Hawaii's FY2012 DSH allotment was also set at $10.0 million, but the allotment was split into two periods. For the first quarter of FY2012 (i.e., October 1, 2011 to December 31, 2011), Hawaii's DSH allotment was $2.5 million. Then, for the remaining three quarters of FY2012, Hawaii's DSH allotment was $7.5 million.

For FY2013 and subsequent years, Hawaii's annual DSH allotment will increase in the same manner applicable to low DSH states. Currently, all states, including low DSH states, receive DSH allotments equal to the prior year's allotment increased by the percent change in CPI-U for the previous fiscal year.

Tennessee

Statute specifies that Tennessee's DSH allotment for each year from FY2007 to FY2011 is the greater of $280.0 million or the federal share of the DSH payments reflected in TennCare[27] for the demonstration year ending in 2006. In accordance with this provision, Tennessee's DSH allotment was $305.4 million (i.e., the federal share of the DSH payments reflected in TennCare for the demonstration year ending in 2006) from FY2007 to FY2011. The statute further limits the amount of federal funds available to Tennessee for DSH payments to 30% of Tennessee's DSH allotment. Under this limit, the federal DSH funding available to Tennessee for each year from FY2007 to FY2011 was $91.6 million (i.e., 30% of $305.4 million).

For the first quarter of FY2012 (i.e., October 1, 2011 through December 31, 2011), Tennessee's DSH allotment was $76.4 million[28] and subject to the 30% limit. For the last three fiscal quarters

---

[25] Section 1115 of the Social Security Act gives the Secretary of Health and Human Services authority to approve experimental, pilot, or demonstration projects that promote the objectives of the Medicaid and CHIP programs.

[26] These laws include the Tax Relief and Health Care Act of 2006 (P.L. 109-432), the Medicare, Medicaid, and SCHIP Extension Act of 2007 (P.L. 110-173), the Medicare Improvements for Patients and Providers Act of 2008 (P.L. 110-275), the Children's Health Insurance Program Reauthorization Act of 2009 (P.L. 111-3), and the Patient Protection and Affordable Care Act (P.L. 111-148 as amended).

[27] TennCare is the name of Tennessee's Medicaid program, which operates under a Section 1115 waiver.

[28] This amount is one-fourth of $305,451,928, which was the DSH allotment for Tennessee for each year from FY2007 to FY2011.

---

of FY2012, Tennessee received a DSH allotment of $47.2 million that was *not* subject to the 30% limit. In total, Tennessee had access to $70.1 million[29] in federal DSH funding in FY2012.

In FY2013, Tennessee will have a DSH allotment of $53.1 million that is *not* subject to the 30% limit. After FY2013, the statute does not provide federal DSH allotments to Tennessee.

Table 3. Federal DSH Funding Available to Tennessee and Hawaii

FY2007 to FY2014

Fiscal Year	Hawaii	Tennessee
FY2007	$10,000,000	$91,635,578
FY2008	$10,000,000	$91,635,578
FY2009	$10,000,000	$91,635,578
FY2010	$10,000,000	$91,635,578
FY2011	$10,000,000	$91,635,578
FY2012	$10,000,000	$70,108,895
FY2013	=$10,000,000 * (% Change in CPI-U for FY2012)	$53,100,000
FY2014	=FY2013 Allotment * (% Change in CPI-U for FY2013)	$0

Source: Section 1923(f)(6) of the Social Security Act; Centers for Medicare & Medicaid Services, "Medicaid Program; Final FY 2009 and Preliminary FY 2011 Disproportionate Share Hospital Allotments, and Final FY 2009 and Preliminary FY 2011 Institutions for Mental Diseases Disproportionate Share Hospital Limits," 76 *Federal Register* 148, January 3, 2011; Centers for Medicare & Medicaid Services, "Medicaid Program; Disproportionate Share Hospital Allotments and Institutions for Mental Diseases Disproportionate Share Hospital Limits for FYs 2010, 2011, and Preliminary FY 2012 Disproportionate Share Hospital Allotments and Limits ," 77 *Federal Register* 43301, July 24, 2012.

Notes: This chart does not provide DSH allotments for Hawaii and Tennessee but the federal DSH funding available to Hawaii and Tennessee. For Hawaii, the DSH allotment and the federal DSH funding available is the same. However, Tennessee's allotment for FY2007 to FY2011 is $305,451,928, but the federal DSH funding available to Tennessee is limited to 30% of the DSH allotment ($305,451,928 * 0.30 = $91,635,578). Tennessee's DSH funding for FY2012 is the combination of $22,908,895 (30% of $76,362,982) for the first fiscal quarter and $47,200,000 for the last three fiscal quarters.

CPI-U = Consumer Price Index for all Urban consumers.

DSH Allotment Reductions

The ACA is expected to reduce the number of uninsured individuals in the United States starting in 2014 through the health insurance coverage provisions (including the ACA Medicaid expansion as impacted by the Supreme Court's ruling). Built on the premise that with fewer uninsured individuals there should be less need for Medicaid DSH payments, the ACA included a provision directing the Secretary of the Department of Health and Human Services (HHS) to make aggregate reductions in Medicaid DSH allotments equal to $500 million in FY2014, $600 million in FY2015, $600 million in FY2016, $1.8 billion in FY2017, $5.0 billion in FY2018, $5.6 billion in FY2019, and $4.0 billion in FY2020.[30] [31]

---

[29] $70,108,895 = $22,908,895 (i.e., 30% of $76,362,982) + $47,200,000

[30] Section 1923(f)(7) of the Social Security Act.

Despite the assumption that reducing the uninsured would reduce the need for Medicaid DSH payments, the ACA was written so that, after the specific reductions for FY2014 through FY2020, DSH allotments would have returned to the amounts states would have received without the enactment of ACA. In other words, in FY2021, states' DSH allotments would have rebounded to their pre-ACA reduced level with the annual inflation adjustments for FY2014 to FY2021.

However, the Middle Class Tax Relief and Job Creation Act of 2012 (P.L. 112-96) extended the FY2020 DSH reduction for an additional year. Specifically, for FY2021, states' DSH allotments will be their FY2020 DSH allotment (as impacted by the aggregate $4.0 billion ACA reduction) increased by the percentage change in CPI-U for FY2020.[32] Under current law, in FY2022, states' DSH allotments will be determined as though the DSH reductions from ACA and the Middle Class Tax Relief and Job Creation Act of 2012 did not occur. In other words, states' DSH allotments will rebound to their pre-ACA reduced levels with the annual inflation adjustments for FY2014 to FY2022.

Figure 1 shows the estimate of aggregate DSH allotments for FY2012 through FY2024 prior to ACA, under ACA, and under current law (i.e., under ACA and the Middle Class Tax Relief and Job Creation Act of 2012). Under current law, the aggregate DSH reductions will be nominal from FY2014 to FY2016. Then, the aggregate reductions will phase up to an estimated 43% reduction in FY2019, and in FY2020 and FY2021, the aggregate DSH reductions will phase down to roughly a 30% reduction. In FY2022, DSH allotments will rebound to the pre-ACA reduced levels.

(...continued)

[31] The United States Supreme Court decision in *National Federation of Independent Business (NFIB) v. Sebelius* (issued June 28, 2012) did not impact this provision of ACA. Only the provision expanding Medicaid eligibility to all nonelderly individuals was impacted by the Supreme Court decision.

[32] Section 1923(f)(8) of the Social Security Act.

Figure 1. Total DSH Allotments Before the Reductions, with the ACA Reductions, and Under Current Law

($ in billions)

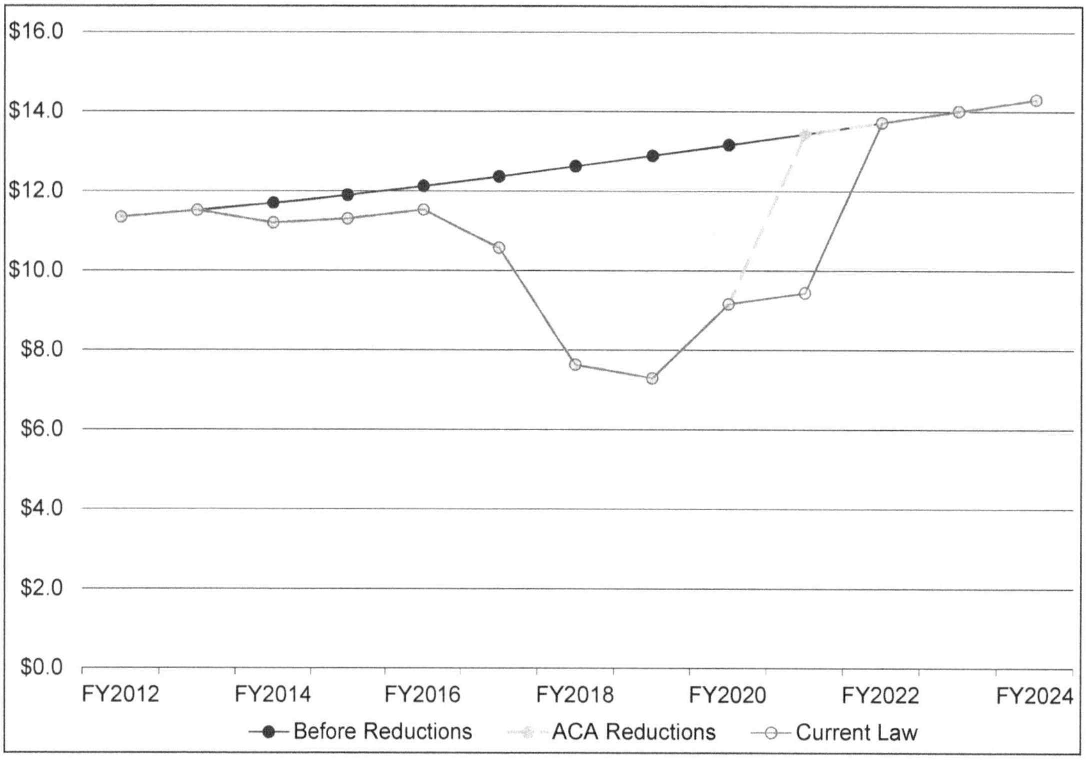

Source: CRS calculation based on preliminary FY2012 DSH allotments.

Note: The CPI-U factor used to inflate the DSH allotments is based on the factors built into the Congressional Budget Office's "The Budget and Economic Outlook: Fiscal Years 2012 to 2022" from January 2012.

Reductions to State DSH Allotments

While the aggregate DSH reduction amounts are specified in statute, the Secretary of HHS is responsible for determining how to distribute the aggregate DSH reductions among the states using some broad statutory guidelines. The Secretary of HHS is required to impose *larger* percentage DSH reductions on states that

- have the lowest percentage of uninsured individuals (determined by the Census Bureau's data, audited hospital cost reports, and other information likely to yield accurate data) during the most recent fiscal year with available data (see **Table B-1** for states' percentage of uninsured) or

- do *not* target their DSH payments to hospitals with high volumes of Medicaid patients and high levels of uncompensated care (excluding bad debt).

The statute also requires the Secretary of HHS to impose *smaller* percentage reductions on low DSH states (i.e., states with total Medicaid DSH payments for FY2000 between 0% and 3% of total Medicaid medical assistance expenditures). In **Appendix B**, **Table B-1** includes the low DSH state designations.

The last specification provided in statute requires the Secretary of HHS to take into account the extent to which the DSH allotment for a state was included in the budget neutrality calculation for a coverage expansion approved under a Section 1115 waiver as of July 31, 2009.

To date, the Secretary of HHS had not issued guidance regarding how the DSH reductions will be applied to each state's DSH allotments. However, on December 10, 2012, CMS issued guidance indicating that HHS will proposed the DSH allotment reduction methodology for public comment early in 2013.[33]

Depending on the methodology chosen by the Secretary of HHS to implement the DSH reductions, in general, states with the lowest percentage of uninsured individuals should receive relatively larger percentage DSH reductions. In addition, states that do not target their DSH payments to hospitals with the most Medicaid patients and highest uncompensated care should receive relatively larger percentage DSH reductions. Also, low DSH states should receive relatively smaller percentage DSH reductions. As a result, a non-low DSH state with a low percent of uninsured individuals that does not target its DSH payments should receive a relatively larger percentage reduction, and a low DSH state with a high percent of uninsured individuals that targets its DSH payments should receive a relatively smaller percentage DSH reduction.

The magnitude of the Medicaid DSH reductions (especially in the later years) is such that most (if not all) states are expected to have DSH allotment reductions. However, states might be able to take action to lessen the magnitude of the Medicaid DSH reductions for their state. States might be able to impact the criteria related to how they target their DSH payments and the percent of uninsured individuals. However, states do not have the ability to impact the last two criteria concerning low-DSH states and Section 1115 waiver budget neutrality calculations.

Furthermore, states' ability to potentially impact the magnitude of their Medicaid DSH reductions depends on whether the Secretary of HHS decides to calculate the distribution of the DSH reductions one time or annually. For instance, if the Secretary decides to calculate the distribution of the DSH reductions annually using up-to-date information, then states that do not currently target their DSH payments could make their DSH payments more targeted in order to lessen the magnitude of their DSH reductions. Though, the Secretary could decide to calculate the distribution of the DSH reductions using information about how states target their DSH payments from one point in time, such as the date ACA was enacted. In this situation, even if states made their DSH payments more targeted, the change would not affect the states' DSH allotment reductions.

States have less control over the percent of uninsured individuals in their state, but if the Secretary of HHS decides to calculate the distribution of DSH reductions annually using up-to-date information, there is potential for states to take action to impact the percent of uninsured individuals in their state in order to influence their DSH reductions. A significant decision available to states that would impact the percent of uninsured individuals in each state is whether or not to implement the ACA Medicaid expansion.

---

[33] Centers for Medicare & Medicaid Services, *Frequently Asked Questions on Exchanges, Market Reforms and Medicaid*, December 10, 2012.

DSH Reductions and the ACA Medicaid Expansion

Without guidance from the Secretary of HHS, it is unclear exactly how the DSH reductions will be distributed among the states. However, it is feasible that states' decisions whether or not to implement the ACA Medicaid expansion could impact the magnitude of states' DSH reductions.

ACA Medicaid Expansion and the Supreme Court

Beginning in 2014 (or sooner at state option), the ACA expands Medicaid to include a new mandatory eligibility group: all adults under age 65 with income up to 133% of the federal poverty level (FPL) (effectively 138% FPL with the modified adjusted gross income[34] 5% FPL income disregard).[35] Originally, it was assumed that all states would implement the ACA Medicaid expansion in 2014 as required by statute because implementing the ACA Medicaid expansion was required in order for states to receive *any* federal Medicaid funding. However, on June 28, 2012, the United States Supreme Court issued its decision in *National Federation of Independent Business (NFIB) v. Sebelius*[36] finding that the federal government cannot terminate the federal Medicaid funding a state receives for its current Medicaid program if a state refuses to implement the ACA Medicaid expansion. If a state accepts the new ACA Medicaid expansion funds, it must abide by the new expansion coverage rules. However, based on the Court's opinion, it appears that a state can refuse to participate in the ACA Medicaid expansion without losing any of its current federal Medicaid matching funds.[37]

The Supreme Court decision only impacts the ACA Medicaid expansion, so the provision reducing Medicaid DSH allotments remains unchanged. This means the Supreme Court ruling does not affect the ACA Medicaid DSH reduction amounts or the statutory criteria the Secretary must use to determine a methodology for distributing the DSH reductions among states. However, the fact that some states may not implement the ACA Medicaid expansion could impact how the DSH reductions are distributed among the states. Specifically, states' decisions whether or not to implement the ACA Medicaid expansion could impact the percentage of uninsured individuals in their state, which is one of the criteria the Secretary must use to determine how to distribute the Medicaid DSH reductions among states.

ACA Expected to Reduce the Percent of Uninsured in All States

The percentage of uninsured individuals in all states is expected to decrease through a combination of ACA health insurance coverage provisions that increase access to health insurance (most of which will be effective starting in 2014). The ACA increases access to health insurance by establishing the health insurance exchanges, which are structured marketplaces for the sale and

---

[34] The modified adjusted gross income (MAGI) is a new income definition used for determining Medicaid income eligibility for certain individuals beginning in 2014. For more information about MAGI, see CRS Report R41997, *Definition of Income in ACA for Certain Medicaid Provisions and Premium Credits*, coordinated by Janemarie Mulvey.

[35] Historically, Medicaid eligibility was generally limited to low-income children, pregnant women, parents of dependent children, the elderly, and people with disabilities. For more information about the ACA changes to Medicaid, see CRS Report R41210, *Medicaid and the State Children's Health Insurance Program (CHIP) Provisions in ACA: Summary and Timeline*, by Evelyne P. Baumrucker et al.

[36] 132 S. Ct. 2566 (2012).

[37] For a discussion of the Supreme Court's decision on the Medicaid expansion, *see* CRS Report R42367, *Medicaid and Federal Grant Conditions After NFIB v. Sebelius: Constitutional Issues and Analysis*, by Kenneth R. Thomas.

purchase of health insurance. Also, certain individuals will be eligible for federal premium cost-sharing subsidies to help them afford health insurance.[38] The other major health insurance coverage provision included in the ACA is the Medicaid expansion.

After the Supreme Court decision, the health insurance exchanges and the premium cost-sharing subsidies are still expected to reduce the percent of uninsured individuals in all states. However, the ACA Medicaid expansion is expected to reduce the number of uninsured individuals by less than previously estimated because some states are expected to decide *not* to implement the ACA Medicaid expansion.

Even if a state does not implement the ACA Medicaid expansion, some of the individuals that would have been covered by the Medicaid expansion may still gain health insurance coverage as a part of the ACA health insurance coverage provisions. The ACA provides premium tax credits and cost-sharing subsidies to individuals with household income between 100% and 400% of the federal poverty level (FPL) that do not have access to minimum essential coverage.[39] As a result, most uninsured individuals with incomes between 100% and 133% (effectively 138%) of FPL living in states that decide *not* to implement the ACA Medicaid expansion may become eligible for these premium tax credits and cost-sharing subsidies to purchase health insurance through the health insurance exchanges.[40]

Regardless of whether a state decides to implement the ACA Medicaid expansion or not, all states could experience an increase in Medicaid enrollment, due to the "woodwork" effect. This is the name for uninsured individuals who are currently eligible but not enrolled in Medicaid enrolling in Medicaid due to increased media attention and outreach efforts. The impact of the woodwork effect depends on the percentage of a state's population that is currently eligible and not enrolled in Medicaid. Estimates find that nationally 7.3 to 9.0 million uninsured children and adults are currently eligible but not enrolled in Medicaid.[41]

How States' Decisions About the ACA Medicaid Expansion Could Impact Their DSH Reductions

Each state's percentage of uninsured individuals will be impacted by the state's decision about the ACA Medicaid expansion. However, states' percentage of uninsured individuals will be impacted

---

[38] For more information about the American Health Benefit Exchanges and the federal subsidies, see CRS Report R42663, *Health Insurance Exchanges Under the Patient Protection and Affordable Care Act (ACA)*, by Bernadette Fernandez and Annie L. Mach.

[39] The definition of minimum essential coverage is broad. It includes Medicare Part A, Medicaid, the State Children's Health Insurance Program (CHIP), Tricare, the TRICARE for Life program, the veteran's health care program, the Peace Corps program, a government plan (local, state, federal) including the Federal Employees Health Benefits Program (FEHBP) and any plan established by an Indian tribal government, any plan offered in the individual, small group or large group market, a grandfathered health plan, and any other health benefits coverage, such as a state health benefits risk pool, as recognized by the Secretary of HHS in coordination with the Treasury Secretary.

[40] Uninsured individuals with household income below 100% of FPL and living in a state that does not implement the ACA Medicaid expansion are not eligible for the premium tax credits or cost-sharing subsidies.

[41] Benevieve M. Kenney, Lisa Dubay, Stephen Zuckerman, and Michael Huntress, *Opting Out of the Medicaid Expansion under the ACA: How Many Uninsured Adults Would not Be Eligible for Medicaid?*, The Urban Institute Health Policy Center, July 5, 2012; Benjamin D. Sommers and Arnold M. Epstein, "Perspective: Why States Are So Miffed about Medicaid - Economics, Politics, and the "Woodwork Effect"," *The New England Journal of Medicine*, vol. 365, no. 2, pp. 100-102.

---

by factors other than the ACA Medicaid expansion. For instance, states' percentage of uninsured individuals will also be impacted by the activity in the health insurance exchanges and changes in employer-sponsored insurance coverage.

States' decisions about whether or not to implement the ACA Medicaid expansion will impact states' percentage of uninsured individuals, which could impact states' Medicaid DSH reductions. However, the magnitude of states' Medicaid DSH reductions depends on a number of factors. As mentioned previously, the statute provides the Secretary of HHS with four criteria to use in determining the allocation of the Medicaid DSH reductions, and states' percentage of uninsured individuals is just one of those criteria.

The extent to which the change in each state's percent of uninsured individuals impacts each state's Medicaid DSH reductions depends on the methodology the Secretary of HHS uses to distribute the DSH reductions among states. For instance, the more weight the Secretary gives the criteria for the percent of uninsured individuals, the more states' decisions about the expansion could impact states' DSH reductions.

In addition, as mentioned previously, the Secretary could calculate the distribution of the DSH reductions one time or annually. If the Secretary chooses to do the calculation one time, then states' decisions whether or not to implement the ACA Medicaid expansion are unlikely to impact the distribution of the Medicaid DSH reductions because the ACA Medicaid expansion begins in January 2014, which is three months after the Medicaid DSH reductions are to begin. However, if the Secretary of HHS chooses to calculate the distribution annually using up-to-date information, then states' decisions about the ACA Medicaid expansion could impact the distribution of the DSH reductions.

How states' decisions regarding the ACA Medicaid expansion impact the allocation of the DSH reductions among states depends on which states decide *not* to implement the expansion and which states decide to implement the expansion. Specifically, state characteristics that could impact the allocation of Medicaid DSH reductions are states' current percentage of uninsured individuals and states' current Medicaid eligibility levels.

If a state that currently has one of the lowest percentages of uninsured individuals chooses *not* to implement the ACA Medicaid expansion, then the percent of uninsured individuals for that state could reduce less than other states that do implement the expansion. Since the measure of percent of uninsured individuals is a relative ranking of states, the state's decision *not* to implement the ACA Medicaid expansion could cause the state's percent of uninsured to go from one of the lowest percentages to an average percentage. States with the lowest percentage of uninsured individuals are supposed to get the largest percentage DSH reductions, which means this state could reduce the magnitude of its DSH allotment reduction by *not* implementing the ACA Medicaid expansion.

Under the Medicaid program, some eligibility groups are mandatory, meaning that all states must cover them; other eligibility groups are optional. As a result of state differences in optional coverage, Medicaid eligibility varies significantly from state to state. If a state with relatively lower levels of Medicaid eligibility chooses to implement the ACA Medicaid expansion, then that state would be expected to lower its percentage of uninsured individuals more than other states implementing the ACA Medicaid expansion. As a result, this state could increase the magnitude of its DSH allotment reduction by implementing the ACA Medicaid expansion.

Since the Supreme Court ruling, some states have stated their intention to implement the ACA Medicaid expansion, other states have asserted that they will not implement the expansion, and most states remain uncommitted. However, it should be noted that states are not locked into their intentions regarding the implementation of the ACA Medicaid expansion. CMS has stated that states face no deadline for deciding when and if they will implement the ACA Medicaid expansion. Also, according to CMS, states can choose to implement the expansion and later drop Medicaid eligibility back to their pre-ACA Medicaid expansion levels.[42]

Lawmakers in six states (Florida, Georgia, Louisiana, Mississippi, South Carolina, and Texas) have publicly stated their state will *not* implement the ACA Medicaid expansion, and five states (Iowa, Maine, Nebraska, Nevada, and New Jersey) have indicated they are leaning towards *not* implementing the expansion.[43] Twelve states (Arkansas, California, Connecticut, Delaware, Hawaii, Illinois, Maryland, Massachusetts, Minnesota, Rhode Island, Vermont, and Washington) and the District of Columbia have indicated they will implement the ACA Medicaid expansion, and two states (Kentucky and Oregon) are leaning toward implementing the expansion.[44] (**Table B-1** shows how each of these states currently ranks with respect to the percentage of uninsured individuals.)[45]

All of the states indicating they will *not* implement the ACA Medicaid expansion currently have relatively high percentages of uninsured individuals and relatively lower Medicaid eligibility levels for nondisabled adults under age 65.[46] Depending on how the Secretary chooses to distribute the Medicaid DSH reductions, by not implementing the ACA Medicaid expansion, these states might be able to reduce the magnitude of their DSH reductions.

While there are some exceptions, most of the states indicating they will implement the ACA Medicaid expansion tend to have relatively lower percentages of uninsured individuals and relatively higher Medicaid eligibility levels for nondisabled adults under age 65.[47] Depending on how the Secretary chooses to distribute the Medicaid DSH reductions, by implementing the ACA Medicaid expansion, these states might increase the magnitude of their DSH reductions.

Again, depending on how the Secretary decides to distribute the DSH reductions among the states, as states' percent of uninsured individuals declines more than other states their percentage of the DSH reductions could increase, and as states' percent of uninsured individuals reduces less than other states their percentage of DSH reductions could decrease. The percent of uninsured individuals for states that do implement the expansion are expected to reduce significantly more than states that do not implement the expansion. As a result, depending on how the Secretary

---

[42] Centers for Medicare & Medicaid Services, *Frequently Asked Questions on Exchanges, Market Reforms and Medicaid*, December 10, 2012.

[43] The Advisory Board Company, *Where Each State Stands on ACA's Medicaid Expansion: A Roundup of What Each State's Leadership Has Said about their Medicaid Plans*, July 5, 2012 (Updated November 8, 2012).

[44] Ibid.

[45] New state elected officials may have been elected in the November 6, 2012 election, and the new elected officials may make different decisions regarding the implementation of the ACA Medicaid expansion. For instance, in Maine, Democrats gained controlled of both houses of the state legislature, and Maine's Democratic leadership has indicated its intention to fully implement the ACA, including the Medicaid expansion. (Phil Galewitz, "Maine May Warm to 'Obamacare' After Democratic Sweep," *Kaiser Health News*, November 8, 2012.)

[46] U.S. Census Bureau, American Community Survey, 2011; Medicaid and CHP Payment and Access Commission, *Report to the Congress on Medicaid and CHIP*, March 2012.

[47] Ibid.

---

administers the DSH reductions, states that choose *not* to implement the ACA Medicaid expansion could have relatively smaller percentage DSH reductions than they otherwise would have had because these states are expected to have relatively larger uninsured populations.

While states' decisions about the ACA Medicaid expansion potential implications for states' Medicaid DSH reductions, states' decisions about whether or not to implement the ACA Medicaid expansion are complicated. The factors states are considering include the state cost of Medicaid coverage for the newly eligible adults; the state cost of the increase in Medicaid coverage for individuals that are currently eligible but not enrolled in Medicaid; potential state savings from current state-funded programs for individuals that will gain Medicaid coverage; and the economic value of additional health care spending for the state economy.[48]

Potential Medicaid DSH reductions are not a significant factor in states' decisions whether or not to implement the ACA Medicaid expansion because the impact of the Medicaid DSH reductions pales in comparison to other potential impacts. For instance, while the aggregate Medicaid DSH reductions from FY2014 to FY2021 total $22 billion, if all states implement the ACA Medicaid expansion it is estimated that all the ACA health insurance coverage provisions would reduce uncompensated care by $183 billion.[49]

Impact on Hospitals

Hospitals are concerned about whether their state will implement the ACA Medicaid expansion because the DSH allotments will be reduced by the same total national amount whether or not states implement the expansion. If a state implements the expansion, the uncompensated care for hospitals should decline along with the DSH allotments (though not proportionally). However, if a state chooses *not* to implement the expansion, the demand for uncompensated hospital care is expected to persist but the amount of Medicaid DSH payments hospitals receive to subsidize such care may be reduced.[50] As a result, hospitals could be expected to encourage states to implement the ACA Medicaid expansion in order to reduce the uncompensated care for hospitals. Even though, Medicaid provider rates are generally lower than the rates paid by private insurance or Medicare, hospitals would rather receive payment from a Medicaid patient than have no payment from an uninsured patient.

DSH Payments

Medicaid state plans must include explanations for how DSH hospitals are defined and how DSH payments are calculated. There are federal requirements that states must follow in making these

---

[48] Deborah Bachrach, *Medicaid Expansion: Factors for State Evaluation*, Presentation at Alliance for Health Reform and Kaiser Family Foundation briefing titled *The Medicaid Expansion: What's at Stake for States?*, November 30, 2012.

[49] John Holahan, Matthew Buettgens, and Caitlin Carroll, et al., *The Cost and Coverage Implications of the ACA Medicaid Expansion: National and State-by-State Analysis*, Kaiser Commission on Medicaid and the Uninsured, Publication #8384, November 2012.

[50] Letter from the Republican Governors Public Policy Committee to President Barack Obama dated July 10, 2012 available at http://www.scribd.com/doc/99730375/Medicaid-and-Exchange-Letter-Final. Sarah Kliff, "The super wonky reason states may join the Medicaid expansion," *The Washington Post*, July 8, 2012. Bob Neal, *The Fiscal and Economic Impacts of Medicaid Expansion in Mississippi, 2014-2025*, Mississippi Public Universities University Research Center, October 2012.

determinations, but for the most part, states are provided significant flexibility in defining DSH hospitals and calculating DSH payments.

Defining DSH Hospitals

The federal government provides states with the following three criteria for identifying DSH hospitals.

- At a minimum, states must provide DSH payments to all hospitals with (1) a Medicaid inpatient utilization rate[51] in excess of one standard deviation[52] above the mean rate for the state or (2) a low-income utilization rate[53] of 25%.

- All DSH hospitals must retain at least two obstetricians with staff privileges willing to serve Medicaid patients.[54]

- A hospital *cannot* be identified as a DSH hospital if its Medicaid utilization rate is below 1%.

As long as states include all hospitals meeting the criteria, states can identify as many or as few hospitals as DSH hospitals. Because of the flexibility, there is a great deal of variation across the states in the proportion and types of hospitals designated as DSH hospitals. Some states target their DSH funds to a few hospitals, while other states provide DSH payments to all the hospitals in the state with Medicaid utilization rates above 1%.[55] For instance, in FY2007, Oregon provided DSH payments to nine out of 58 hospitals, and New Jersey provided DSH payments to all of the hospitals in the state.[56]

Calculating DSH Payments

States are also provided a good deal of flexibility in terms of the formulas and methods they use to distribute DSH funds among DSH hospitals. The federal government provides minimum and maximum payment criteria, but otherwise federal law does not address the specific payment amounts states should provide to each DSH hospital.

---

[51] The formula for the Medicaid utilization rate is the number of days of care furnished to Medicaid beneficiaries during a given period divided by the total number of days of care provided during the period. (Section 1923(b)(2) of the Social Security Act).

[52] The "standard deviation" is a statistical measure of the dispersion of hospitals' utilization rates around the average; the use of this measure identifies hospitals whose Medicaid utilization is unusually high.

[53] The formula for the low-income utilization rate is the sum of two fractions. The first fraction is total Medicaid revenue for services plus other payments from state and local governments divided by the total amount of hospital revenue for patient services. The second fraction is the total amount of hospital charges for inpatient hospital services minus the total amount of revenue from state and local governments divided by total hospital charges. (Section 1923(b)(3) of the Social Security Act).

[54] There are exceptions to this rule for children's hospitals, hospitals that do not offer non-emergency obstetric services, and certain rural hospitals. (Section 1923(d) of the Social Security Act).

[55] Courtney Burke, "Health Reform: Uncompensated Care Costs and Reductions In Medicaid DSH Payments," *Health Affairs Blog*, October 15, 2010.

[56] CRS review of DSH annual reports and the American Hospital Association Hospital Statistics (2012 Edition).

States must make minimum payments to DSH hospitals using one of three methodologies:[57]

- the Medicare DSH methodology,[58]

- a formula providing Medicaid DSH payments that increase in proportion to the percentage by which the hospital's Medicaid inpatient utilization rate exceeds one standard deviation above the mean, or

- a formula that varies DSH payments according to the type of hospitals.[59]

DSH payments to individual hospitals are subject to a cap.[60] This hospital-specific limit prohibits DSH payments from being greater than 100% of the cost of providing inpatient and outpatient services to Medicaid and uninsured patients less payments received from Medicaid and uninsured patients.[61]

The Definition of Uninsured

Under the hospital-specific DSH limit, uninsured is defined in the statute as individuals who "have no health insurance (or other source of third-party coverage) for the services furnished during the year."[62] In the past, CMS has provided conflicting guidance regarding this definition, and, in January 2012, CMS issued a proposed rule to address this issue.[63]

The hospital-specific limit was implemented through the Omnibus Reconciliation Act of 1993 (P.L. 103-66), and, following the passage of the law, CMS did not issue a rule. However, CMS did issue a State Medicaid Director Letter delineating the agency's interpretation of the statute, which stated that individuals who have no health insurance (or other third party coverage) for the

---

[57] Section 1923(c) of the Social Security Act.

[58] Medicare DSH funds are paid to qualifying hospitals through an adjustment within the applicable prospective payment system (PPS). Generally, DSH hospitals receive the additional payments based on a DSH patient percentage (DPP) which is calculated by adding the proportion of a hospital's Medicare inpatient days provided to poor Medicare beneficiaries (those who receive Supplemental Security Income or SSI) to the proportion of total hospital days provided to Medicaid recipients. A few urban acute care hospitals receive DSH payments under an alternative formula. An acute care hospital will not receive operating DSH payments unless its low-income patient share or DPP exceeds 15%. After that minimum threshold of 15% is met, the size of a hospital's DSH adjustment will vary by the hospital's bed size, urban or rural location, or whether it receives special treatment as a rural referral center (RRC). Under the current operating DSH thresholds and formulas, the DSH adjustment that a small urban or rural hospital can receive is capped at 12%, while large (100 beds and more) urban hospitals, large rural hospitals (500 beds and more), and RRCs can receive an uncapped adjustment that can be significantly greater.

[59] If a state chooses to reimburse according to the type of hospital, the state must ensure that all hospitals of each type are treated equally and payments are reasonably related to the hospitals' Medicaid or low-income patient cost, volume, or proportion of Medicaid or low-income patients.

[60] Section 1923(g) of the Social Security Act.

[61] In California, the hospital-specific cap for public hospitals is 175% of the unreimbursed costs. California's hospital-specific DSH cap for public hospitals was established in the Balanced Budget Act of 1997 (P.L. 105-33) and made permanent by the Medicare, Medicaid, and SCHIP Balanced Budget Refinement Act of 1999 (which was included in the Consolidated Appropriations Act of 2000, P.L. 106-113).

[62] Section 1923(g)(1)(A) of the Social Security Act.

[63] Department of Health and Human Services' Centers for Medicare & Medicaid, "Medicaid Program; Disproportionate Share Hospital Payments - Uninsured Definition," 77 *Federal Register* 2500, January 18, 2012.

---

services provided during the year include those "who do not possess health insurance which applies to the service for which the individual sought treatment."[64]

This interpretation remained in effect until the January 19, 2009, which was the effective date for the 2008 DSH final rule implementing the DSH auditing and reporting requirements (these requirements are discussed later in the report in the section titled "State Reporting and Auditing Requirements").[65] In promulgating the 2008 DSH final rule, CMS defined "uninsured" as individuals who do not have a legally liable third party payer for hospital services.[66] The 2008 DSH final rule relied on the existing regulatory definition of creditable coverage developed to implement the Health Insurance Portability and Accountability Act of 1996 (P.L. 104-191). The definition of uninsured from the 2008 final rule superseded the guidance from the 1994 State Medicaid Director Letter.

Concerns were raised about the new definition of uninsured because this definition appeared to exclude from uncompensated care (for Medicaid DSH purposes) the costs of many services that were provided to individuals with creditable coverage but were outside the scope of such coverage. For instance, the definition excluded individuals who exhausted their insurance benefits and who reached lifetime insurance limits for certain services, as well as services not covered in a benefit package.

In response to these concerns, CMS issued a proposed rule on January 18, 2012 that would change the definition of uninsured for Medicaid DSH purposes to a service-specific definition. The proposed definition would require a determination of whether, for each specific service furnished during the year, the individual has third party coverage. As a result, under the proposed definition, the following services would be included services not within a covered benefit package and services beyond the annual and lifetime limits.[67]

Institutions for Mental Disease (IMD) DSH Limits

Federal statute limits the amount of DSH payments for IMDs[68] and other mental health facilities.[69] DSH payments to IMDs and other mental health facilities above the state-specific dollar limit are not eligible for federal matching funds.

Each state receives an IMD DSH limit that is the lesser of:

---

[64] State Medicaid Directors letter, August 17, 1994.

[65] The reporting requirements originally established in the Balanced Budget Act of 1997 (P.L. 105-33) were extended by the Medicare Prescription Drug, Improvement, and Modernization Act of 2003 (MMA, P.L. 108-173).

[66] Department of Health and Human Services' Centers for Medicare & Medicaid Services, "Medicaid Program: Disproportionate Share Hospital Payments," 73 *Federal Register* 77904, December 19, 2008.

[67] Department of Health and Human Services' Centers for Medicare & Medicaid, "Medicaid Program; Disproportionate Share Hospital Payments - Uninsured Definition," 77 *Federal Register* 2500, January 18, 2012.

[68] An "institution for mental diseases" is defined as "a hospital, nursing facility, or other institution of more than 16 beds, that is primarily engaged in providing diagnosis, treatment, or care of persons with mental diseases, including medical attention, nursing care and related services." (Section 1905(i) of the Social Security Act)

[69] Section 1923(h) of the Social Security Act.

- a state's FY1995 total IMD and other mental health facility DSH expenditures (i.e., including both state and federal spending) applicable to the state's FY1995 DSH allotment as reported on the Form CMS-64 as of January 1, 1997 or

- the amount equal to the product of the state's current year total DSH allotment and the applicable percentage, which is the lesser of 33% or the percent of FY1995 DSH expenditures that went to mental health facilities.

The IMD DSH limits fit within the state DSH allotments. In other words, when DSH payments to hospitals and IMDs and other mental health facilities are summed together, the total is required to be less than or equal to the state's DSH allotments in **Table 2**.

As with the DSH allotments, the IMD DSH limits are published in periodic *Federal Register* notices. In **Appendix C**, **Table C-1** includes each state's preliminary IMD DSH limit for FY2012.

DSH Expenditures

The implementation of the DSH allotments effectively controlled the significant growth of DSH expenditures from the early 1990s. As shown in **Figure 2**, total Medicaid DSH expenditures (i.e., including both federal and state expenditures) have remained relatively stable since the implementation of the federal DSH allotments in FY1993. In FY2011, DSH expenditures totaled $17.3 billion, and the federal share of those payments was $9.8 billion.

Figure 2. Total Medicaid DSH Expenditures, FY1990-FY2011 Estimate

($ in billions)

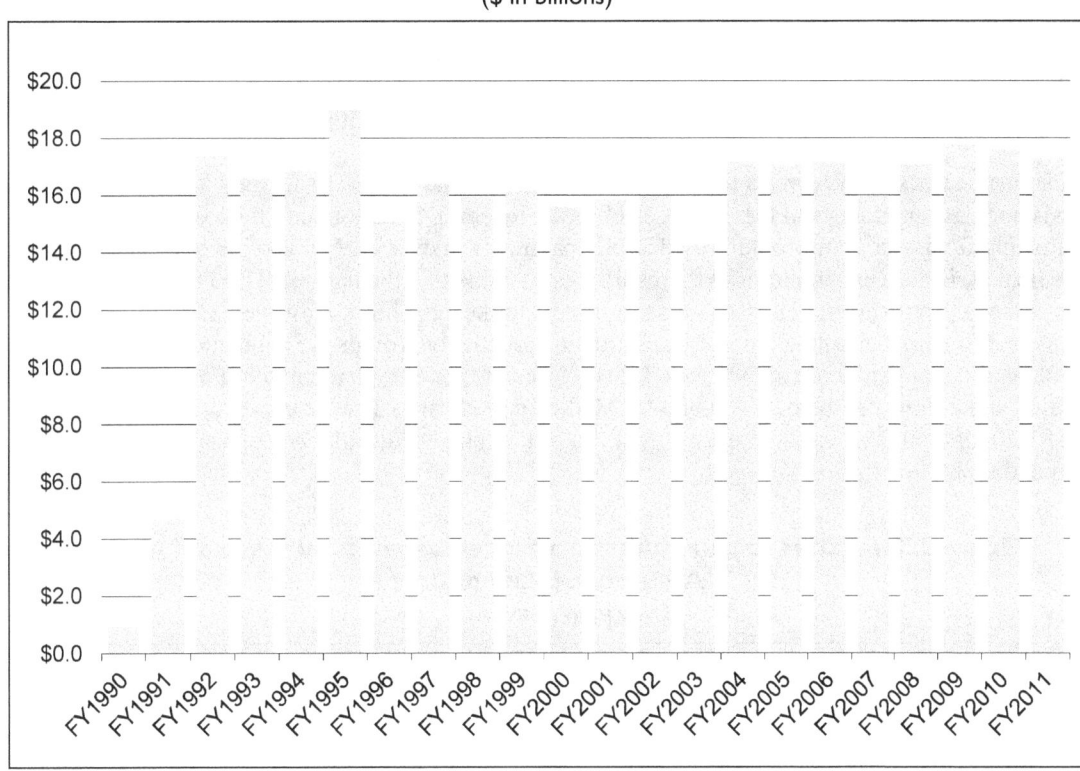

Source: Payments estimated by the Urban Institute for FY1990-FY1992; data from CMS for FY1993-FY1996; CMS-64 data for FY1997-FY2011.

Note: Total Medicaid DSH expenditures include both federal and state spending and payments to both hospitals and institutions for mental disease.

While Medicaid DSH expenditures have been relatively stable, total Medicaid medical assistance expenditures (i.e., including federal and state expenditures and excluding expenditures on administrative activities) have generally grown at a rate faster than the economy as measured by the gross domestic product for the period of FY1990 to FY2011.

The law establishing DSH allotments (i.e., Medicaid Voluntary Contribution and Provider-Specific Tax Amendments of 1991, P.L. 102-234) specified a national DSH payment limit equal to 12% of the total amount of Medicaid medical assistance spending (i.e., including federal and state expenditures and excluding expenditures for administrative activities) for all 50 states and the District of Columbia.[70] This is a target but not an absolute cap.

The national DSH payment limit is different from the 12% limit on state DSH allotments because the 12% national payment limit restricts both federal and state spending while the 12% limit for allotments caps only federal spending. The national DSH payment target states that aggregate DSH payments (including federal and state expenditures) should not be more than 12% of the

---

[70] 42 C.F.R. § 447.297.

total amount of Medicaid medical assistance expenditures for all 50 states and the District of Columbia. The federal statute limits state DSH allotments (i.e., the maximum amount of Medicaid DSH federal funds) to no more than 12% of each state's total Medicaid medical assistance expenditures (i.e., including federal and states expenditures but excluding administrative expenditures), which means the federal share of DSH expenditures cannot be more than 12% of each state's total Medicaid medical assistance expenditures.

This means if a state receives a federal DSH allotment equal to 12% of its total Medicaid medical assistance expenditures and the state uses all of its federal DSH allotment, then with the state matching funds, the state would provide DSH payments in excess of 12% of its total Medicaid medical assistance expenditures. As a result, it is possible that the national DSH target could be surpassed even if state DSH allotments are subject to the 12% limit. However, as shown in **Figure 3**, the implementation of DSH allotments effectively brought DSH payments under the 12% national target within a few years. DSH allotments were implemented in FY1993, and total DSH expenditures fell below 12% of total Medicaid medical assistance expenditures in FY1996. In FY2012, total DSH expenditures were 4.2% of the total Medicaid medical assistance expenditures.

Figure 3. Total DSH Expenditures as a Percentage of Total Medicaid Medical Assistance Expenditures

FY1990 to FY2011

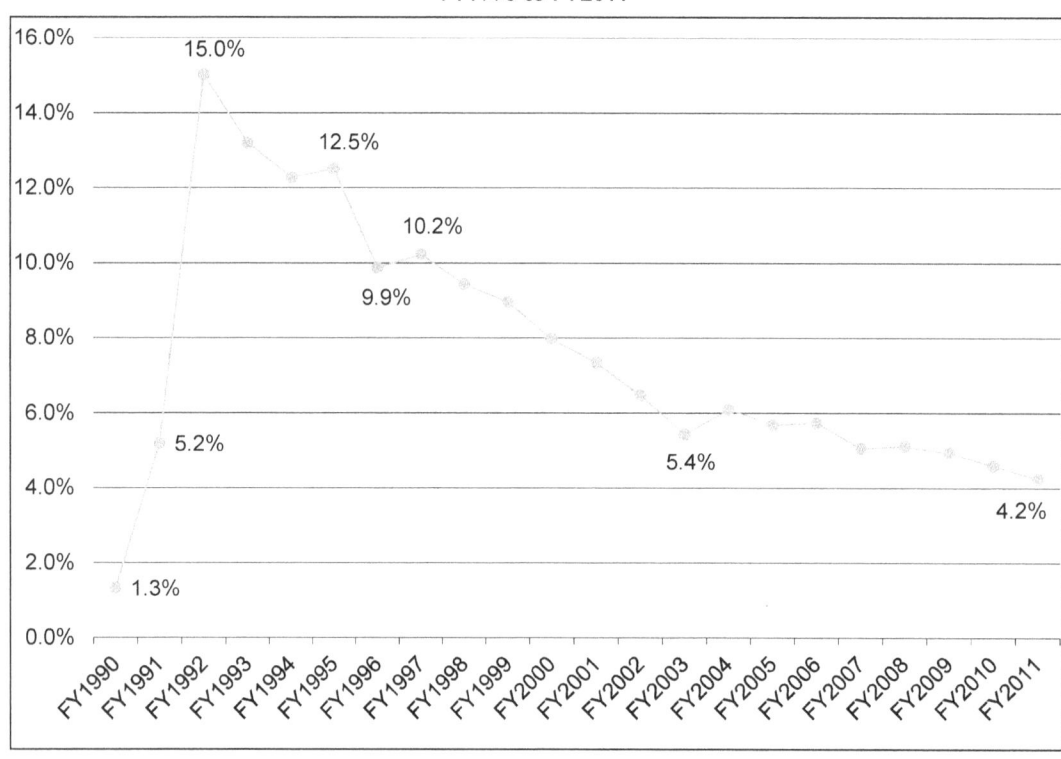

Sources: CRS calculation using DSH payment estimates from the Urban Institute for FY1990-FY1992; DSH payment data from Centers for Medicare & Medicaid Services (CMS) for FY1993-FY1996; DSH payment data for FY1997-FY2011 and medical assistance expenditure data for FY1990-FY2011 from Form CMS-64 data.

Note: Total DSH expenditures and total Medicaid medical assistance expenditures (i.e., excluding expenditures for administrative activities) include both the federal and state expenditures.

DSH expenditures are highly concentrated in a few states. As shown in **Figure 4**, five states (New York, California, Texas, New Jersey, and Pennsylvania) accounted for more than half of the FY2011 DSH expenditures, and ten states accounted for over two-thirds of all DSH expenditures. It makes sense that some of these states (New York, California, Texas, New Jersey, Pennsylvania, and Ohio) accounted for a large portion of the total Medicaid DSH expenditures because these states were among the top ten highest spending states in terms of total medical assistance expenditures (i.e., including federal and state expenditures and excluding expenditures for administrative activities) for FY2011. On the other hand, Missouri, Louisiana, South Carolina, and Alabama ranked 15th, 22nd, 25th, and 26th (respectively) in terms of total medical assistance expenditures (i.e., including federal and state expenditures and excluding expenditures for administrative activities) for FY2011, but these states were among the top ten highest Medicaid expenditures states. This means, Missouri, Louisiana, South Carolina, and Alabama spend a larger proportion of their Medicaid budget on Medicaid DSH payments relative to most other states.[71]

Figure 4. States' Share of Total Medicaid DSH Expenditures

FY2011

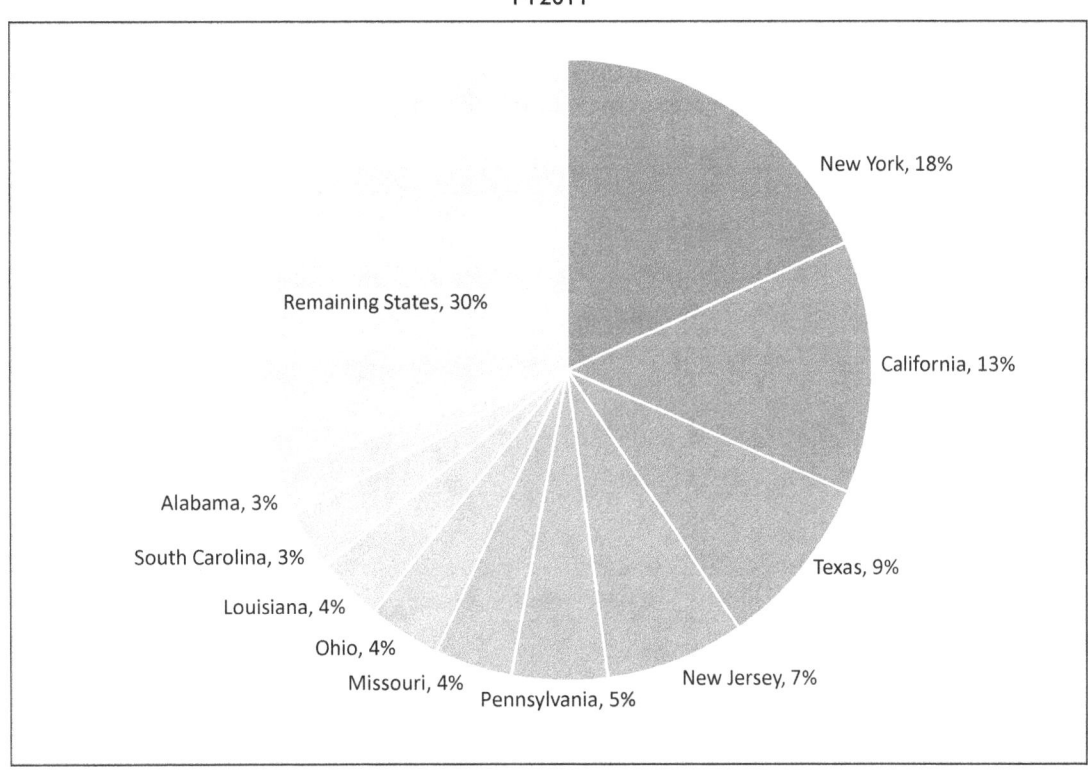

Source: CRS calculation using Centers for Medicare & Medicaid Services' Form CMS-64 data from FY2011.

Notes: The states included in the "remaining states" category had DSH expenditures that accounted for less than 3% of total DSH expenditures. In **Appendix D**, **Table D-1** shows state-by-state DSH spending.

---

[71] In FY2011, only New Jersey and New Hampshire spent a larger proportion of their Medicaid budget (i.e., Medicaid DSH payments as a percentage of medical assistance expenditures) than Missouri, Louisiana, South Carolina, and Alabama.

State Variation

As mentioned previously, there is significant variation among the states in how each state DSH program is structured, and there is also variation from state to state with respect to DSH expenditures. Two distinct differences are (1) the percent of a state's total Medicaid medical assistance expenditures (i.e., including federal and state expenditures and excluding expenditures for administrative activities) a state's DSH expenditures account for and (2) the proportion of DSH payments going to hospitals versus IMDs.

DSH as a Percentage of Total Medical Assistance Expenditures

Figure 5 shows FY2011 total DSH expenditures (i.e., including both federal and state expenditures) as a percentage of total Medicaid medical assistance expenditures (i.e., including federal and state expenditures and excluding expenditures for administrative activities). DSH expenditures made in FY2011 ranged from 0.1% of total Medicaid medical assistance expenditures in South Dakota and Wyoming to 12.1% in New Jersey.

Figure 5. Total State DSH Expenditures as a Percentage of Total Medicaid Medical Assistance Expenditures

FY2011

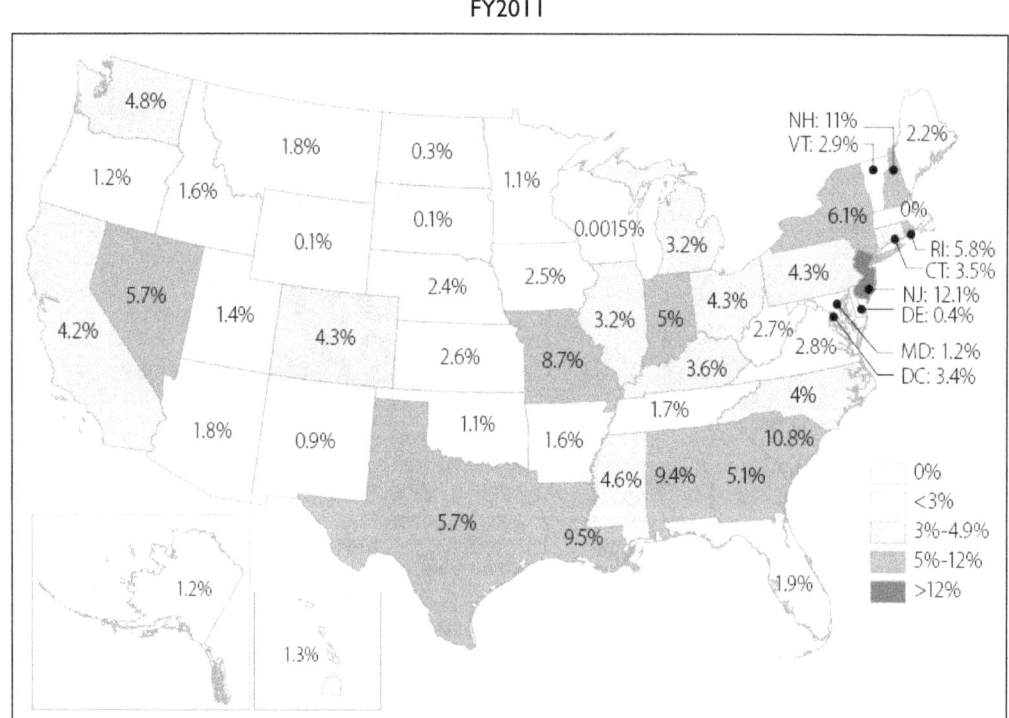

Source: CRS calculation using Centers for Medicare & Medicaid Services' Form CMS-64 data for FY2011,

Note: Total DSH expenditures and total Medicaid medical assistance expenditures (i.e., excluding expenditures for administrative activities) include both the federal and state share of expenditures.

Massachusetts does not have DSH expenditures because Massachusetts' Section 1115 waiver allows the state to use its DSH allotment to fund the state's Health Safety Net which reduces the number of uninsured in Massachusetts. In **Appendix D**, **Table D-1** shows each state's total DSH expenditures and total Medicaid medical assistance expenditures.

In FY2011, one state (New Jersey) had DSH expenditures in excess of 12% of total Medicaid medical assistance expenditures,[72] which was the threshold used to determine "high" DSH states when DSH allotments were first implemented.[73] This is down from FY1993, when 21 states were considered "high" DSH states.

Hospital Versus IMD

Nationally, 83% of DSH expenditures are allocated to hospitals, and the remaining 17% is distributed to IMDs and other mental health facilities. This distribution varies by state. As shown in **Figure 6**, in FY2011, most states targeted their DSH expenditures to hospitals, with fifteen states[74] allocating all of their DSH expenditures to hospitals. Other states focused their DSH expenditures on IMDs and other mental health facilities. Three states (South Dakota, Maine, and Delaware) made all of their DSH expenditures to IMDs and other mental health facilities.

---

[72] The 12% limit on DSH allotments caps the federal share of DSH expenditures to no more than 12% of a state's total Medicaid medical assistance expenditures. However, when the federal DSH allotment funds are matched with the state share of the Medicaid DSH payments, a state could provide DSH payments in excess of 12% of its total Medicaid medical assistance expenditures.

[73] When DSH allotments were first implemented, states with DSH expenditures greater than 12% of their total Medicaid medical assistance expenditures were classified as "high-DSH" states, and "high-DSH" states did not receive annual increases to their DSH allotment.

[74] The fifteen states allocating all of their DSH expenditures to hospitals are Colorado, Georgia, Hawaii, Idaho, Iowa, Mississippi, Montana, Nebraska, Nevada, Rhode Island, Tennessee, Utah, Vermont, Wisconsin, and Wyoming.

Figure 6. Proportion of State DSH Expenditures Allocated to Hospitals and IMDs
FY2011

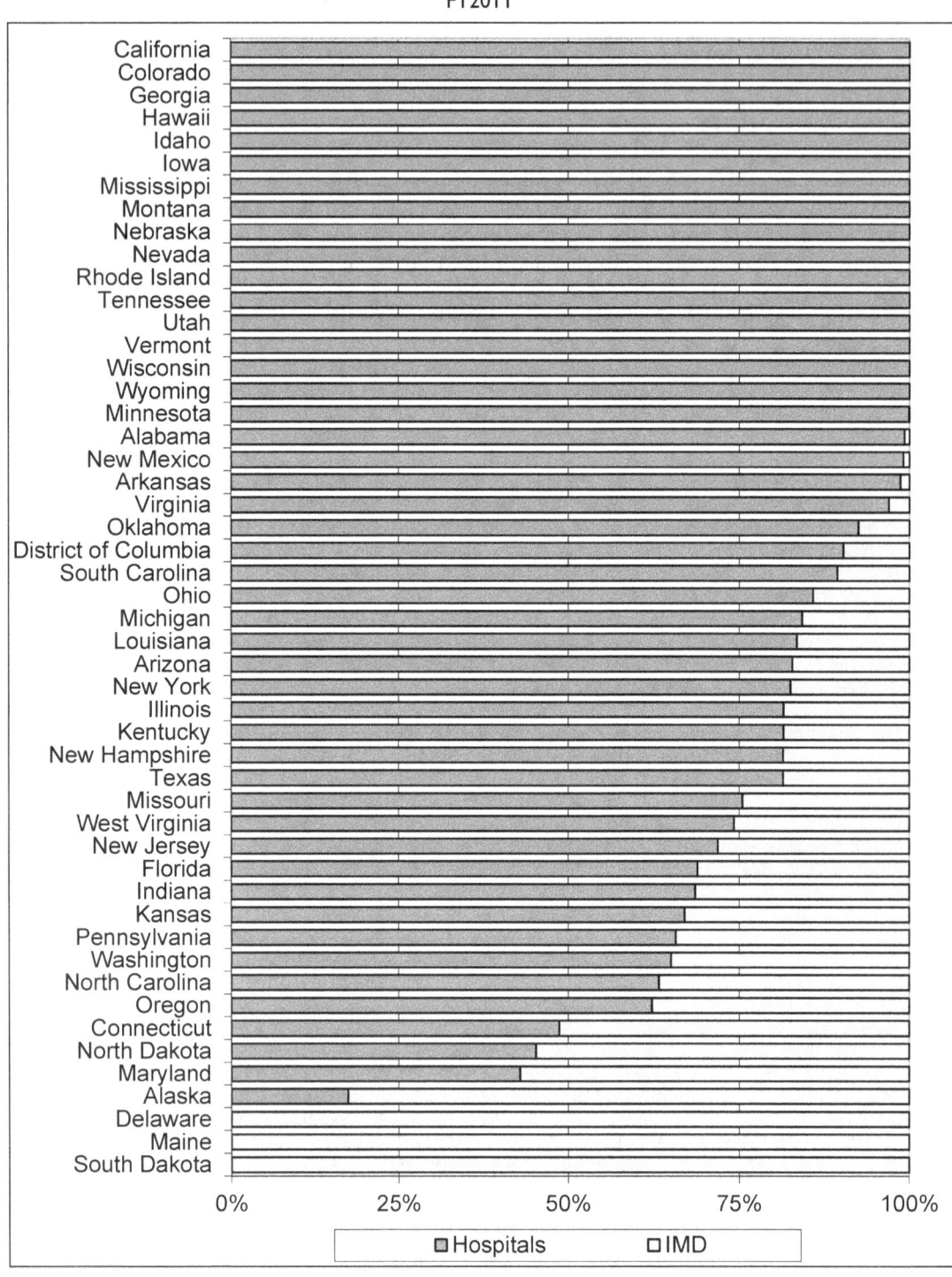

Source: CRS calculation using Centers for Medicare & Medicaid Services' Form CMS-64 data from FY2011.

Notes: Table D-1 shows each state's hospital and IMD DSH expenditures.

IMD = Institutions for Mental Diseases and other mental health facilities.

State Reporting and Auditing Requirements

Since FY1993, each state has been required to provide quarterly reports with information about the aggregate DSH payments made to hospitals. Then, in 1997 and again in 2003, Congress enhanced the DSH reporting requirements in response to HHS Office of the Inspector General audits and Government Accountability Office reports detailing state violations in the DSH program.

The Balanced Budget Act of 1997 (BBA, P.L. 105-33) required states to provide an annual report to the Secretary of HHS describing the method used to target DSH funds and to calculate DSH payments. Then, in 2003, MMA mandated that beginning in state plan rate year[75] (SPRY) 2005, states were required to submit annual reports and independently certified audits.[76]

States' annual DSH reports must provide detailed information about each hospital receiving a DSH payment. For each hospital, the report must include the following information: the hospital-specific DSH limit, the Medicaid inpatient utilization rate, the low income utilization rate, state-defined DSH qualification criteria, Medicaid basic payments, other supplemental payments, total Medicaid uncompensated care, total uninsured uncompensated care, federal Section 1011 payments,[77] and DSH payments.

The annual independent certified audits must verify that hospitals retain the DSH payment; DSH payments are made in accordance with the hospital-specific DSH limits; uncompensated care only includes inpatient and outpatient services; and the state separately documented and retains records of DSH payments (including the methodology for calculating each hospital's DSH payments).

The annual independent certified audits must be completed by the last day of the federal fiscal year ending three years from the end of the SPRY under audit. The annual DSH reports are due at the same time as the independent certified audits. If a state does not submit the independent certified audit by this deadline, the state could lose the federal DSH matching funds for the SPRYs subsequent to the date the audit is due.[78]

To ensure a period for developing and refining the reporting and auditing techniques, findings of state reports and audits for SPRY2005 to SPRY2010 will not be given weight except to the extent that the findings draw into question the reasonableness of the state uncompensated care cost estimates used for calculations of prospective DSH payments. For SPRY2011 and after, audit

---

[75] Medicaid state plan rate year means the 12-month period defined by a state's approved Medicaid state plan in which the state estimates eligible uncompensated care costs and determines corresponding DSH payments as well as all other Medicaid payment rates. The period usually corresponds with the state's fiscal year or the federal fiscal year but can correspond to any 12-month period defined by the state as the Medicaid state plan rate year.

[76] Section 1923(j) of the Social Security Act.

[77] Under Section 1011 of MMA, hospitals, physicians, and ambulance service providers are eligible for Section 1011 payments for services furnished to the following types of patients: undocumented aliens; aliens who have been paroled into a United States port of entry for the purpose of receiving eligible services; and Mexican citizens permitted to enter the United States on a laser visa, issued in accordance with the requirements of regulations prescribed under the Immigration and Nationality Act. (Centers for Medicare & Medicaid Services, *Section 1011: Fact Sheet Federal Reimbursement of Emergency Health Services Furnished to Undocumented Alien.*)

[78] 42 CFR 455.304(a).

---

findings demonstrating that DSH payments exceed the hospital-specific cost limit will be regarded as discovery of overpayment to providers. This will require the state to return the federal share of the overpayment to the federal government (unless the DSH payments are redistributed to other qualifying hospitals).[79]

Conclusion

Since DSH allotments were implemented in FY1993, DSH payments have remained relatively stable. Over the same period of time, Medicaid medical assistance expenditures have generally grown at a rate faster than the economy (as measured by the gross domestic product). As a result, total DSH expenditures have dropped as a percentage of total Medicaid medical assistance expenditures from 15.0% in FY1992 to 4.2% in FY2011.

Over the next few years, DSH expenditures will continue to decline as a percentage of Medicaid medical assistance expenditures due to the ACA DSH reductions. The impact of these reductions will vary by state according to the uninsurance rate of each state; whether a state is a "low DSH state"; and, how a state targets its DSH payments.

Currently, the DSH reductions are slated to end in FY2021 with state DSH allotments returning to the level states would have received without the DSH reduction for FY2022 and subsequent years. However, the future of Medicaid DSH payments is uncertain. Congress may decide to extend the DSH reductions, as Congress did with the Middle Class Tax Relief and Job Creation Act of 2012 (P.L. 112-96). Also, as states build experience with the ACA Medicaid expansion, the role of DSH in Medicaid may be revisited and modified by Congress.

---

[79] Department of Health and Human Services, Centers for Medicare & Medicaid Services, "Medicaid Program; Disproportionate Share Hospital Payments," 73 *Federal Register* 77904, December 19, 2008.

Appendix A. A Chronology of State DSH Allotments Calculations

The Medicaid Voluntary Contribution and Provider-Specific Tax Amendments of 1991 (P.L. 102-234) established ceilings on federal Medicaid DSH funding for each state. Since FY1993, each state has had its own DSH limit, which is referred to as "DSH allotments." These allotments are calculated by the Centers for Medicare & Medicaid Services (CMS) and promulgated in the *Federal Register*. The methodology for calculating these allotments has changed a number of times over the years, and these different methodologies are described below.[80]

FY1993

The original state DSH allotments provided in FY1993 were based on each state's FY1992 DSH payments. This resulted in funding inequities because states that had been providing relatively more DSH payments to hospitals in FY1992 locked in higher Medicaid DSH allotments (and vice versa). As a result, the DSH allotment a state receives is not entirely based on the number of DSH hospitals in the state or the hospital services provided in DSH hospitals to low-income patients.

FY1994 to FY1997

The DSH allotments for FY1994 to FY1997 were based on each state's prior year DSH allotment. The annual growth for each state's DSH allotment depended on whether a state was classified as a "high-DSH" or "low-DSH" state. States with DSH expenditures greater than 12% of their total Medicaid medical assistance expenditures (i.e., federal and state Medicaid expenditures excluding expenditures for administrative activities) were classified as "high-DSH" states, and "high-DSH" states did not receive an increase to their DSH allotment. States with DSH expenditures less than 12% of their total Medicaid medical assistance expenditures were classified as "low-DSH" states, and the growth factor for the DSH allotment for "low-DSH" states was the projected percentage increase for each state's total Medicaid expenditures (i.e., including federal and state spending) for the current year. However, "low-DSH" states' DSH allotments could not exceed 12% of each state's total medical assistance expenditures.[81]

FY1998 to FY2000

Provisions included in the Balance Budget Act of 1997 (BBA, P.L. 105-33) reduced Medicaid DSH expenditures by replacing the state DSH allotment calculations with *fixed* state DSH allotments specified in statute for FY1998 through FY2002.[82] The aggregate fixed allotments for FY1998 totaled $10.3 billion, which was a 50% decrease from the aggregate FY1997 DSH allotments. The aggregate allotments for FY1999 and FY2000 decreased to $10.0 billion and $9.3 billion respectively.

---

[80] Tennessee and Hawaii have had special statutory arrangements for their federal DSH funding since FY2007.

[81] The definition of "low-DSH" state has changed over the years.

[82] Section 1923(f)(2) of the Social Security Act.

Adjustments for Specific States

A number of legislative adjustments were made to the BBA fixed DSH allotments. The Departments of Labor, Health and Human Services, and Education, and Related Agencies Appropriations Act, 1998 (P.L. 105-78) increased the FY1998 DSH allotments for Minnesota and Wyoming. The Omnibus Consolidated and Emergency Supplemental Appropriations Act, 1999 (P.L. 105-277) increased the FY1999 DSH allotments for Minnesota, New Mexico, and Wyoming. The Medicare, Medicaid, and SCHIP Balanced Budget Refinement Act of 1999 (included in the Consolidated Appropriations Act 2000, P.L. 106-113) increased the FY2000, FY2001, and FY2002 DSH allotments for the District of Columbia, Minnesota, New Mexico, and Wyoming.

FY2001 and FY2002

The fixed state allotments were supposed to last through FY2002 with the aggregate DSH allotments slated to decrease in FY2001 and again in FY2002. However, the Medicare, Medicaid, and SCHIP Benefits Improvement and Protection Act of 2000 (BIPA, which was incorporated into the Consolidated Appropriations Act of 2001, P.L. 106-554) eliminated the DSH reductions for FY2001 and FY2002 and provided states with increases to their DSH allotments. Specifically, the DSH allotments for those two years were determined by increasing each state's prior year DSH allotment by the percent change in the Consumer Price Index for all Urban Consumers (CPI-U) for the prior fiscal year. These state DSH allotments could not exceed 12% of a state's total medical assistance expenditures for the allotment year. This is referred to as the 12% rule.[83]

Extremely Low DSH States

BIPA also established a special rule for DSH allotments for "extremely low DSH states," which were defined as states with FY1999 DSH expenditures greater than 0% and less than 1% of total Medicaid medical assistance expenditures (i.e., federal and state Medicaid expenditures excluding expenditures for administrative activities).[84] The FY2001 DSH allotments for extremely low DSH states were increased to 1% of the each state's FY2001 total medical assistance expenditures. Then, the FY2002 DSH allotments for extremely low DSH states was each state's FY2001 DSH allotment increased by the percentage change in CPI-U for FY2001, subject to the 12% rule.[85]

FY2003

For non-extremely low DSH states, FY2003 DSH allotments were each state's FY2002 fixed DSH allotment determined in BBA (i.e., not states' actual DSH allotment for FY2002 as provided by BIPA) increased by the percent change in CPI-U for FY2002, subject to the 12% rule. For most states, the FY2002 state DSH allotments provided by BBA were less than the actual state allotments states received in FY2002. As a result, in general, FY2003 DSH allotments were lower

---

[83] Department of Health and Human Services' Center for Medicare & Medicaid Services, "Medicaid Program; Disproportionate Share Hospital Payments," 69 *Federal Register* 15850, March 26, 2004.

[84] Ten states were classified as extremely low DSH states for FY2001 and FY2002: Arkansas, Idaho, Iowa, Montana, Nebraska, North Dakota, South Dakota, Utah, Virginia, and Wisconsin.

[85] Department of Health and Human Services' Center for Medicare & Medicaid Services, "Medicaid Program; Disproportionate Share Hospital Payments," 69 *Federal Register* 15850, March 26, 2004.

than the allotments states received in FY2002.[86] This was not the case for extremely low DSH states, which received FY2003 DSH allotments based on their actual FY2002 DSH allotment increased by percentage change in CPI-U for FY2002.[87]

FY2004

The Medicare Prescription Drug, Improvement, and Modernization Act of 2003 (MMA, P.L. 108-173) addressed the drop in DSH allotments for many states from FY2002 to FY2003 by exempting FY2002 DSH allotment amounts from the 12% rule and providing a 16% increase in DSH allotments for FY2004.

Low DSH States

MMA also discontinued the special arrangement for extremely low DSH states and instead established low DSH states—defined as those states in which total DSH payments for FY2000 were less than 3% of the state's total Medicaid medical assistance expenditures. For such states, FY2004 DSH allotments were each state's FY2003 DSH allotment increased by 16%.

After FY2004

State DSH allotments for years after FY2004 are set to be equal to each state's FY2004 DSH allotment, unless a state's allotment as determined by the calculation in place prior to MMA would equal or exceed the FY2004 allotment for that state. For any years a state's DSH allotments would be higher under the pre-MMA calculation, that state's DSH allotment will be equal to its DSH allotment from the prior fiscal year increased by the percentage change in the CPI-U for the prior fiscal year, subject to the 12% rule.[88]

Low DSH States

By statute, the definition of low DSH state is a state with FY2000 DSH expenditures greater than 0% but less that 3% of total Medicaid medical assistance expenditures for FY2000. So states determined to be low DSH states in FY2004 continue to be low DSH states regardless of the states' DSH expenditures in years after FY2000.

For FY2004 through FY2008, low DSH states received DSH allotments in each year equal to each state's prior year DSH allotment increased by 16%, subject to the 12% rule. For FY2009 forward, the allotment for low DSH states is equal to the prior year allotment amount increased by the percentage change in the CPI-U (subject to the 12% rule), which is the same DSH increase provided to non-low DSH states.

---

[86] This is referred to as the "DSH dip."

[87] Department of Health and Human Services' Center for Medicare & Medicaid Services, "Medicaid Program; Disproportionate Share Hospital Payments," 69 *Federal Register* 15850, March 26, 2004.

[88] Ibid.

District of Columbia

The Deficit Reduction Act of 2005 (DRA, P.L. 109-171) increased the fixed DSH allotments for the District of Columbia for FY2000, FY2001, and FY2002 from $32 million to $49 million. This change was effective as of October 1, 2005. Increasing the District of Columbia's DSH allotments for FY2000 to FY2002 was done for the purposes of determining the District of Columbia's FY2006 DSH allotment. This change made the District of Columbia's DSH allotment for FY2006 $57.7 million, which was a $20.0 million increase over what the District of Columbia would have gotten without the change. The provision took effect on October 1, 2005 and applies to FY2006 and subsequent fiscal years.

FY2009 and FY2010

The American Recovery and Reinvestment Act of 2009 (ARRA, P.L. 111-5) temporarily increased states' DSH allotments for FY2009 and FY2010.[89] Specifically, ARRA provided states with a FY2009 DSH allotment that was 102.5% of the FY2009 allotment states would have received without ARRA. Then, states' FY2010 DSH allotments were 102.5% of each state's FY2009 DSH allotment as determined under ARRA. For both years, the ARRA DSH provisions were not applied to the DSH allotments for states that would have had a higher DSH allotment as determined without application of the ARRA DSH provisions. After FY2010, states' annual DSH allotments returned to being determined as they were prior to the enactment of ARRA.[90]

---

[89] The ARRA increase to DSH allotments did not apply to the allotments for Hawaii and Tennessee.

[90] Section 5001(e) of ARRA specifies that the ARRA temporary increase to the FMAP does not apply to DSH payments.

Appendix B. ACA DSH Reductions

Under the Patient Protection and Affordable Care Act (ACA, P.L. 111-148 as amended), it is expected that the ACA health insurance coverage expansions will reduce the number of uninsured individuals served by hospitals starting in 2014. For this reason, theoretically, there will be less need for DSH payments. As a result, the ACA directs the Secretary of the Department of Health and Human Services (HHS) to make aggregate reductions in Medicaid DSH allotments from FY2014 through FY2020.[91]

To achieve these aggregate reductions, the Secretary will be required to impose the *largest* percentage reductions on states that

- have the lowest percentage of uninsured individuals (determined on the basis of data from the Bureau of the Census, audited hospital cost reports, and other information likely to yield accurate data) during the most recent fiscal year with available data or

- do not target their DSH payments to hospitals with high volumes of Medicaid patients, and hospitals that have high levels of uncompensated care (excluding bad debt).

ACA also requires the Secretary of HHS to impose *smaller* percentage reduction on low DSH states as defined in Section 1923(f)(5)(B) of the Social Security Act. Low DSH states are those states where total Medicaid DSH payments (including federal and state share) for FY2000 were between 0% and 3% of total Medicaid medical assistance expenditures (i.e., including Medicaid spending on health care and excluding expenditures for administrative activities).

Table B-1 shows each state's percentage of uninsured ranked from highest to lowest. The table also indicates low DSH state designations. The information in the table is the most recent data available, and the DSH reductions will not necessarily be determined using the 2011 data.

Depending on the methodology chosen by the Secretary of HHS to implement the DSH reductions, in general, states with the lowest percentage of uninsured individuals should receive larger percentage DSH reductions. Also, low DSH states should receive smaller percentage DSH reductions. Again, depending on how the Secretary decides to implement the DSH reductions, as states' percent of uninsured individuals increases or decreases relative to other states, due to implementing or not implementing the ACA Medicaid expansion among other reasons, states percentage of the DSH reductions could increase or decrease accordingly.

Regardless of whether a state decides to implement the ACA Medicaid expansion or not, all states could experience a reduction in the percentage of uninsured individuals, due to the woodwork effect. This is the name for uninsured individuals that are currently eligible but not enrolled in Medicaid coming out of the woodwork to enroll in Medicaid due to increased media attention and outreach efforts. The impact of the woodwork effect depends on the percentage of a state's population that is currently eligible and not enrolled in Medicaid. Estimate finds that, nationally,

---

[91] The FY2020 DSH reduction was extended to FY2021 through the Middle Class Tax Relief and Job Creation Act of 2012 (P.L. 112-96). Specifically, for FY2021, states' DSH allotments will be their FY2020 DSH allotment (as impacted by the aggregate $4.0 billion ACA reduction) increased by the percentage change in CPI-U for FY2020.

7.3 to 9.0 million uninsured children and adults are currently eligible but not enrolled in Medicaid.[92]

Similarly, the uninsured population for all states is expected to decline as new individuals purchase private health insurance, as the American Health Benefit Exchanges and federal subsidies become available in 2014.[93]

Table B-1. State Factors for DSH Reductions—Percentage of Uninsured Individuals and Low DSH State Designation

State	Percent Uninsured, 2011	Rank for Percent Uninsured	Low DSH State
Texas	23.0%	1	
Nevada	21.9%	2	
Florida	20.9%	3	
Alaska	20.1%	4	X
New Mexico	19.8%	5	X
Georgia	19.6%	6	
Oklahoma	18.7%	7	X
Montana	18.3%	8	X
California	18.1%	9	
Mississippi	17.7%	10	
Louisiana	17.5%	11	
Arizona	17.2%	12	
Arkansas	17.1%	13	X
South Carolina	16.7%	14	
Idaho	16.5%	15	X
North Carolina	16.3%	16	
Oregon	15.7%	17	X
Wyoming	15.4%	18	X
Utah	15.3%	19	X
Colorado	15.1%	20	
West Virginia	14.9%	21	
Tennessee	14.6%	22	

[92] Benevieve M. Kenney, Lisa Dubay, Stephen Zuckerman, and Michael Huntress, *Opting Out of the Medicaid Expansion under the ACA: How Many Uninsured Adults Would not Be Eligible for Medicaid?*, The Urban Institute Health Policy Center, July 5, 2012; Benjamin D. Sommers and Arnold M. Epstein, "Perspective: Why States Are So Miffed about Medicaid - Economics, Politics, and the "Woodwork Effect"," *The New England Journal of Medicine*, vol. 365, no. 2, pp. 100-102.

[93] For more information about the American Health Benefit Exchanges and the federal subsidies, see CRS Report R42663, *Health Insurance Exchanges Under the Patient Protection and Affordable Care Act (ACA)*, by Bernadette Fernandez and Annie L. Mach.

State	Percent Uninsured, 2011	Rank for Percent Uninsured	Low DSH State
Indiana	14.5%	23	
Kentucky	14.4%	24	
Alabama	14.3%	25	
Washington	14.2%	26	
Missouri	13.7%	27	
Illinois	13.1%	28	
New Jersey	13.1%	28	
Kansas	12.6%	30	
Virginia	12.5%	31	
Ohio	11.9%	32	
South Dakota	11.9%	32	X
Michigan	11.8%	34	
Nebraska	11.4%	35	X
New York	11.4%	35	
Rhode Island	10.8%	37	
Maine	10.7%	38	
New Hampshire	10.5%	39	
Maryland	10.4%	40	
Pennsylvania	10.1%	41	
North Dakota	9.8%	42	X
Delaware	9.4%	43	X
Wisconsin	9.0%	44	X
Iowa	8.9%	45	X
Connecticut	8.8%	46	
Minnesota	8.8%	46	X
Hawaii	7.1%	48	
District of Columbia	6.9%	49	
Vermont	6.6%	50	
Massachusetts	4.3%	51	

Source: U.S. Census Bureau, American Community Survey, 2011; Department of Health and Human Services, "Medicaid Program: Disproportionate Share Hospital Allotments and Institutions for Mental Diseases Disproportionate Share Hospital Limits for FYs 2010, 2011, and Preliminary FY 2012 Disproportionate Share Hospital Allotments and Limits ," 77 *Federal Register* 43301, July 24, 2012.

Note: DSH = Disproportionate Share Hospital.

Appendix C. IMD DSH Limits

Under Sections 1923(h) of the Social Security Act, states cannot collect Medicaid federal matching funds for DSH payments to IMDs and other mental health facilities that are in excess of state-specific aggregate limits. The aggregate limit for each state is the lesser of a state's FY1995 DSH expenditures to IMDs and other mental health facilities or the amount equal to the product of a state's current year DSH allotment and the applicable percentage (i.e., the percentage of FY1995 DSH expenditures paid to IMDs and other mental health facilities with a maximum of 33%). **Table C-1** shows states' preliminary IMD DSH limits for FY2012.

Table C-1. States' Preliminary IMD DSH Limits

FY2012

State	IMD DSH Limit
Alabama	$3,054,805
Alaska	$6,883,889
Arizona	$19,163,608
Arkansas	$579,363
California	$777,960
Colorado	$297,388
Connecticut	$52,786,863
Delaware	$3,059,506
District of Columbia	$4,581,595
Florida	$67,589,520
Georgia	$0
Hawaii	$0
Idaho	$0
Illinois	$44,704,138
Indiana	$72,236,300
Iowa	$0
Kansas	$13,940,339
Kentucky	$26,651,979
Louisiana	$80,310,122
Maine	$35,484,498
Maryland	$25,768,504
Massachusetts	$52,817,527
Michigan	$89,556,114
Minnesota	$2,628,607
Mississippi	$0
Missouri	$131,490,365
Montana	$0

State	IMD DSH Limit
Nebraska	$1,025,941
Nevada	$0
New Hampshire	$47,376,974
New Jersey	$178,685,231
New Mexico	$176,720
New York	$302,500,000
North Carolina	$99,694,542
North Dakota	$547,617
Ohio	$59,937,114
Oklahoma	$2,090,951
Oregon	$12,566,330
Pennsylvania	$189,673,090
Rhode Island	$1,249,751
South Carolina	$50,626,422
South Dakota	$444,243
Tennessee	$0
Texas	$170,301,413
Utah	$663,463
Vermont	$5,223,253
Virginia	$3,885,134
Washington	$62,520,306
West Virginia	$13,715,772
Wisconsin	$2,719,014
Wyoming	$0
Total	**$1,939,986,271**

Source: Department of Health and Human Services, "Medicaid Program: Disproportionate Share Hospital Allotments and Institutions for Mental Diseases Disproportionate Share Hospital Limits for FYs 2010, 2011, and Preliminary FY 2012 Disproportionate Share Hospital Allotments and Limits ," 77 Federal Register 43301, July 24, 2012.

Notes: DSH = Disproportionate Share Hospital. IMD = Institutions for Mental Diseases.

Appendix D. State-by-State DSH Expenditures

There is significant variation from state to state with respect to DSH expenditures. Two distinct differences are (1) the proportion of DSH payments going to hospitals and IMDs and (2) total DSH payments as a percent of total Medicaid medical assistance expenditures (i.e., including federal and state expenditures and excluding expenditures for administrative activities).

Nationally, 83% of Medicaid DSH expenditures are allocated to hospitals, and the remaining 17% is distributed to IMDs and other mental health facilities. This distribution varies by state. As shown in **Table D-1**, in FY2011, most states targeted their DSH expenditures to hospitals with fifteen states allocating all of their DSH expenditures to hospitals. However, some states focused their DSH expenditures on IMDs and other mental health facilities. Three states (South Dakota, Maine, and Delaware) used all of their DSH expenditures for IMDs and other mental health facilities.

Table D-1 also shows FY2011 total DSH expenditures (i.e., including both federal and state expenditures) as a percentage of total Medicaid medical assistance expenditures (i.e., including federal and state expenditures and excluding expenditures for administrative activities). DSH expenditures made in FY2011 ranged from 0.1% of total Medicaid medical assistance expenditures in South Dakota and Wyoming to 12.1% in New Jersey.

Table D-1. DSH Expenditures by Type and DSH Expenditures as a Percentage of Medical Assistance Expenditures

FY2011

($ in millions)

State	DSH Expenditures			Total Medical Assistance	DSH Payments as a Percentage of Medical Assistance Expenditures
	Hospital	IMD	Total		
Alabama	$445.8	$3.3	$449.1	$4,793.2	9.4%
Alaska	2.6	12.6	15.2	1,290.5	1.2%
Arizona	137.3	28.5	165.8	8,988.4	1.8%
Arkansas	61.2	0.8	62.0	3,951.8	1.6%
California	2,274.9	0.3	2,275.3	54,305.8	4.2%
Colorado	185.0	0.0	185.0	4,349.0	4.3%
Connecticut	98.1	103.3	201.4	5,812.4	3.5%
Delaware	0.0	5.6	5.6	1,391.7	0.4%
District of Columbia	66.2	7.1	73.3	2,129.5	3.4%
Florida	241.2	108.9	350.1	18,127.9	1.9%
Georgia	410.1	0.0	410.1	8,064.6	5.1%
Hawaii	20.0	0.0	20.0	1,523.9	1.3%
Idaho	24.7	0.0	24.7	1,514.7	1.6%

State	DSH Expenditures			Total Medical Assistance	DSH Payments as a Percentage of Medical Assistance Expenditures
	Hospital	**IMD**	**Total**		
Illinois	334.2	75.7	409.8	12,836.0	3.2%
Indiana	223.9	102.8	326.7	6,566.4	5.0%
Iowa	81.9	0.0	81.9	3,317.1	2.5%
Kansas	46.8	23.1	69.9	2,669.2	2.6%
Kentucky	165.4	37.4	202.8	5,652.1	3.6%
Louisiana	501.0	99.2	600.2	6,297.5	9.5%
Maine	0.0	51.5	51.5	2,356.2	2.2%
Maryland	38.0	50.4	88.4	7,319.5	1.2%
Massachusetts	0.0	0.0	0.0	13,007.4	0.0%
Michigan	326.8	61.1	387.9	12,062.9	3.2%
Minnesota	89.3	0.1	89.4	8,271.2	1.1%
Mississippi	204.1	0.0	204.1	4,410.8	4.6%
Missouri	528.2	171.4	699.6	8,011.2	8.7%
Montana	17.0	0.0	17.0	954.5	1.8%
Nebraska	38.5	0.0	38.5	1,637.3	2.4%
Nevada	88.4	0.0	88.4	1,562.9	5.7%
New Hampshire	121.1	27.5	148.6	1,348.2	11.0%
New Jersey	912.5	357.4	1,269.9	10,501.1	12.1%
New Mexico	28.9	0.3	29.1	3,317.6	0.9%
New York	2,606.7	551.5	3,158.2	51,711.7	6.1%
North Carolina	258.5	150.5	408.9	10,297.1	4.0%
North Dakota	0.8	1.0	1.8	701.9	0.3%
Ohio	569.5	93.4	662.9	15,533.3	4.3%
Oklahoma	40.7	3.3	44.0	4,008.3	1.1%
Oregon	32.9	20.0	52.9	4,386.3	1.2%
Pennsylvania	571.4	297.9	869.3	20,395.0	4.3%
Rhode Island	122.7	0.0	122.7	2,098.7	5.8%
South Carolina	474.6	56.1	530.7	4,930.8	10.8%
South Dakota	0.0	0.5	0.5	750.2	0.1%
Tennessee	139.2	0.0	139.2	7,970.0	1.7%
Texas	1,286.6	292.5	1,579.1	27,847.4	5.7%
Utah	24.0	0.0	24.0	1,733.3	1.4%
Vermont	37.4	0.0	37.4	1,281.9	2.9%
Virginia	189.4	5.9	195.3	6,893.8	2.8%

State	DSH Expenditures			Total Medical Assistance	DSH Payments as a Percentage of Medical Assistance Expenditures
	Hospital	IMD	Total		
Washington	226.7	122.1	348.9	7,335.0	4.8%
West Virginia	54.4	18.9	73.3	2,740.2	2.7%
Wisconsin	0.1	0.0	0.1	6,878.4	0.0%
Wyoming	0.8	0.0	0.8	527.2	0.1%
Total	$14,349.6	$2,941.7	$17,291.3	$408,148.0	4.2%

Source: CRS calculation using Centers for Medicare & Medicaid Services' Form CMS-64 Data for FY2011.

Notes: Medicaid medical assistance expenditures exclude administrative expenditures.

DSH = Disproportionate Share Hospital. IMD = Institutions for Mental Diseases.

a. Massachusetts does not have DSH expenditures because Massachusetts' Section 1115 waiver allows the state to use its DSH allotment to fund the state's Health Safety Net, which is used to offset uncompensated care hospital costs, to pay for designated state health programs, and to subsidize premiums for Commonwealth Care (a program that provides sliding-scale premium subsidies for private health plan coverage for uninsured persons at or below 300% of the federal poverty level).

Author Contact Information

Alison Mitchell
Analyst in Health Care Financing
amitchell@crs.loc.gov, 7-0152